EC made easy

Your Key to Understanding EC, EM, and LS

Second Edition

MW01560187

The Joint Commission

Joint Commission Resources

Environment of Care
Emergency Management
Life Safety

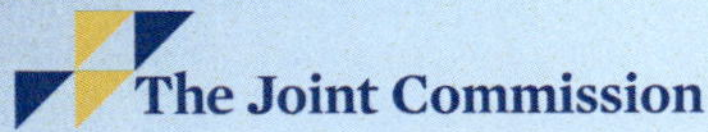
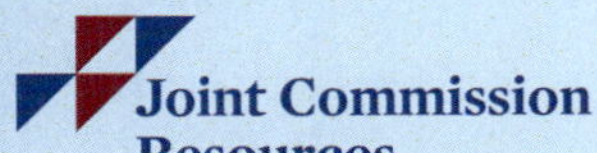

Senior Editor: Holly E. Vossel

Project Manager: Lisa M. King

Content Development Manager: Lisa K. Abel

Editorial Intern: Andrea L. Goethals

Associate Director, Publications: Helen M. Fry, MA

Associate Director, Production and Meeting Support: Johanna Harris

Executive Director, Global Publishing: Catherine Chopp Hinckley, MA, PhD

The Joint Commission/Joint Commission Resources Reviewers: Lynne Bergero, MHSA; Helen M. Fry, MA; Lisa Hardesty, MA, CHSP, HEM, CFI; Caroline Heskett, MPH; James Kendig, MS, CHSP, CHCM, HEM, LHRM; Carrie Mayer, MBA; Kenneth A. Monroe, PE, MBA, CHC, PMP; and Kathy Tolomeo, CHEM, CHSP.

Joint Commission Resources Mission

The mission of Joint Commission Resources (JCR) is to continuously improve the safety and quality of health care in the United States and in the international community through the provision of education, publications, consultation, and evaluation services.

Joint Commission Resources educational programs and publications support, but are separate from, the accreditation activities of The Joint Commission. Attendees at Joint Commission Resources educational programs and purchasers of Joint Commission Resources publications receive no special consideration or treatment in, or confidential information about, the accreditation process.

The inclusion of an organization name, product, or service in a Joint Commission Resources publication should not be construed as an endorsement of such organization, product, or service, nor is failure to include an organization name, product, or service to be construed as disapproval.

This publication is designed to provide accurate and authoritative information in regard to the subject matter covered. Every attempt has been made to ensure accuracy at the time of publication; however, please note that laws, regulations, and standards are subject to change. Please also note that some of the examples in this publication are specific to the laws and regulations of the locality of the facility. The information and examples in this publication are provided with the understanding that the publisher is not engaged in providing medical, legal, or other professional advice. If any such assistance is desired, the services of a competent professional person should be sought.

ISBN: 978-1-59940-993-1 (E-book)
ISBN: 978-1-59940-992-4 (Soft cover)

Library of Congress Control Number: 2015931003

For more information about Joint Commission Resources, please visit http://www.jcrinc.com.

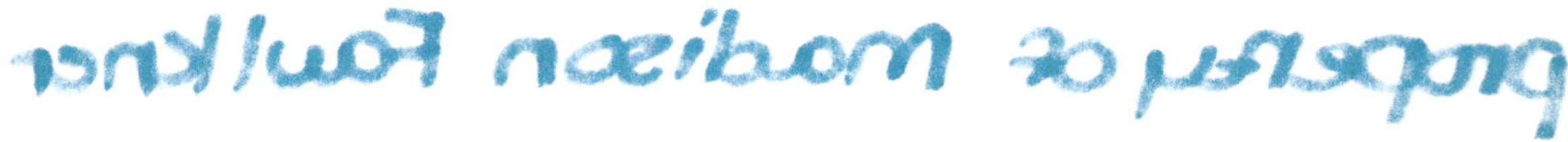

Table of Contents

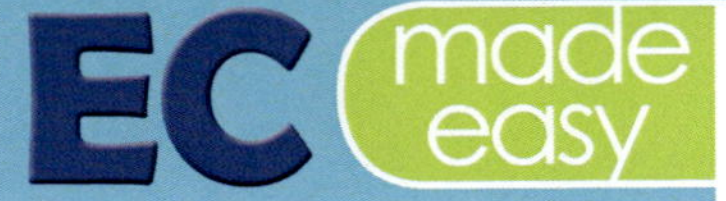

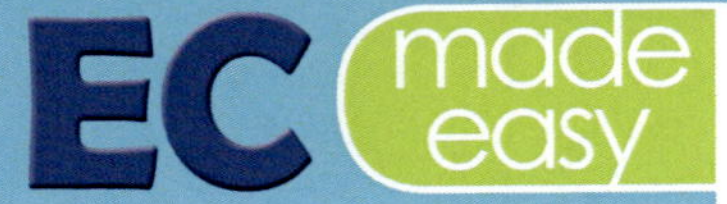

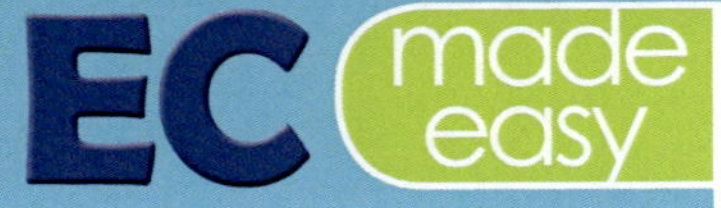

Table of Terms

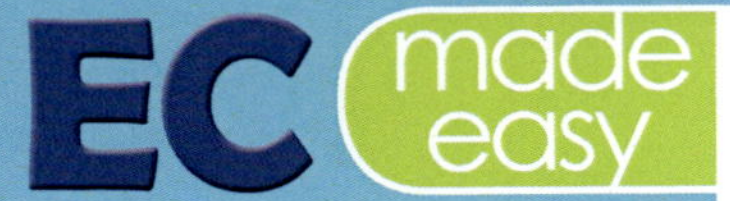

Term	Page	Related Key Concept	Chapter
emergency power supply system (EPSS) and stored emergency power supply system (SEPSS)	110	Utility Systems: Emergency Power Supply System	6
environmental tour	26	Environmental Tours	2
environment of care	2	Responsibility for the Environment of Care	1
equivalency	140	Statement of Conditions™	7
ergonomics	38	Worker Safety	3
evidence-based design (EBD)	174	Planning and Design	9
Evidence of Standards Compliance (ESC)	137	Statement of Conditions™	7
	195	After the Survey	10
exercise	158	Emergency Response Exercises	8
fire rating	126	Life Safety	7
fire safety	118	Fire Safety vs. Life Safety	7
Focused Standards Assessment (FSA)	199	Continuous Compliance	10
hazardous materials	66	Hazmat Inventory	5
hazardous waste	66	Hazmat Inventory	5
hazard vulnerability analysis (HVA)	144	Hazard Vulnerability Analysis	8
hazmat manifest	80	Hazardous Waste Disposal	5
high reliability organization (HRO)	37	General Safety	3
high-risk equipment	87	Medical Equipment: Managing the Program	6
horizontal evacuation	134	"Defend in Place" and the Unit Concept	7
human factors	88	Medical Equipment: Managing the Program	6
Immediate Threat to Health or Safety	191	The Survey Analysis for Evaluating Risk™ (SAFER™) Matrix	10
incident command system (ICS)	154	Incident Command System	8
Information Collection and Evaluation System (ICES)	30	Improvement and ICES	2
interim life safety measures (ILSMs)	138	Statement of Conditions™	7
	175	Managing Construction Risks	9
Intracycle Monitoring (ICM)	198	Continuous Compliance	10

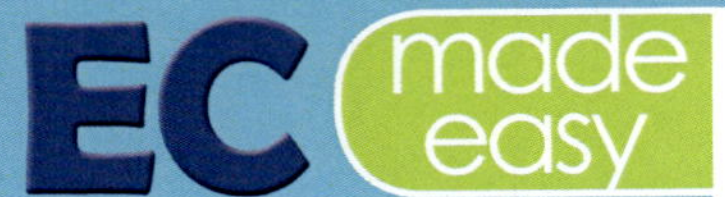

Term	Page	Related Key Concept	Chapter
Requirement for Improvement (RFI)	194	After the Survey	10
response	147	The Four Phases of Emergency Management	8
risk	2	Responsibility for the Environment of Care	1
risk assessment	20	EC Risk Assessments	2
root cause analysis	23	EC Risk Assessments	2
safety	36	General Safety	3
safety and health management system (SHMS)	36	General Safety	3
safety data sheet (SDS)	79	Labeling and Safety Data Sheets	5
safety officer	2	Responsibility for the Environment of Care	1
security-sensitive areas	49	Access Control	4
sentinel event	23	EC Risk Assessments	2
sharps	40	Infection in the Environment	3
	76	Managing Specific Types of Materials	5
smoke compartment	134	"Defend in Place" and the Unit Concept	7
Survey-Related Plan for Improvement (SPFI)	137	Statement of Conditions™	7
	194	After the Survey	10
time-limited waiver (TLW)	197	After the Survey	10
tracer	186	The On-Site Survey Process	10
unit concept	133	"Defend in Place" and the Unit Concept	7
utility map	105	Utility Systems: Managing the Program	6
utility systems	103	Utility Systems: Managing the Program	6
workarounds	39	Worker Safety	3
workplace violence	55	Workplace Violence	4

Introduction

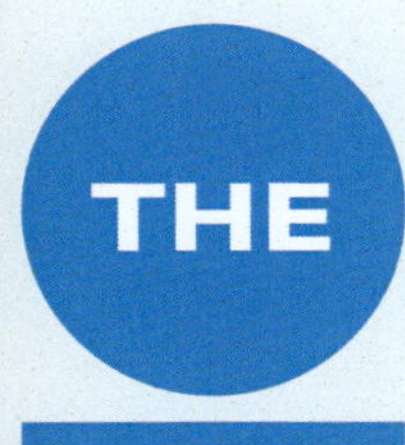

The physical environment of a health care organization is known as the environment of care. It may sound broad and vague. It is broad, covering everything from emergency power to door latches to facility security. But it's not vague; it's actually very specific and detail-oriented. Getting your head around all the details is a challenge. And if you're reading this book, you're probably trying to do that because you're involved in some way in managing the environment of care. We want to help make it easy for you.

This Book Is for You

This book is aimed at four major audiences: accreditation professionals, safety professionals, new facilities directors, and leadership at various levels.

You're an accreditation professional: You're charged with overseeing overall Joint Commission compliance. You're good with understanding the standards related to clinical areas; you most likely came from a clinical background after all. But the complexities of the environment of care can be confusing. This book explains complicated environment of care concepts in plain English. It supports you in your role of dealing with challenging standards and significant safety compliance issues.

You're a safety professional: You maintain a safe environment in your organization by assessing potential hazards or risks, evaluating and implementing preventive measures, and ensuring preparation for emergency response plans. This book

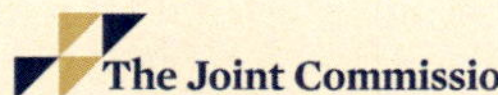

The Joint Commission accredits and certifies more than 21,000 health care organizations and programs in the United States. Joint Commission accreditation and certification is recognized nationwide as a symbol of quality that reflects your organization's commitment to meeting certain performance standards.

helps you understand compliance to help your health care organization provide a safe environment for patients and staff.

You're a new facilities director: Maybe you attained this position because you excelled in some related position in your organization—you were a staff electrician, clinical engineer, or security officer. Or maybe you moved up through the environment of care ranks in your organization, and now you're in charge of the whole operation. In that case, you may know at least some of the Joint Commission compliance–related issues. Or maybe you came out of another industry. So you might know how regulatory compliance works in that industry. This book helps you make sense of compliance in your health care organization. That will help put you in a better position to provide safe and effective care and welcome surveyors who check to see that you do.

You're in a leadership position: Your facilities director is telling you the building needs a new boiler and that the last possible patches have been made to the one you have. But it'll cost big bucks to purchase a new one. How can you make sure that you provide the resources that are truly needed—as opposed to those that are merely wanted? How can you make sure you understand that situation and myriad others like it? Or maybe you're a leader on the front line and you just don't know what's expected of you regarding fire drills, workplace violence, or the intersection of infection control and the environment of care. This book gives you the background to prepare for and understand conversations with your facilities staff and accreditation professionals. It gives you confidence in the decisions you need to make regarding your physical facilities and clinical protocols.

You're working together: Not only is this book for all of you independently; it's for all of you to use together to communicate and collaborate better in your efforts to devise appropriate and effective accreditation compliance strategies—together.

- **Accreditation professionals:** You can sit down with experienced facilities directors to go over concepts in the book and enhance your mutual understanding of those concepts. You can use it to translate environment of care information for clinicians and leadership.

- **Safety professionals:** You can use it to help identify and manage risks related to the physical environment.
- **New facilities directors:** You can use it to learn environment of care concepts and then communicate those to accreditation professionals or leadership.
- **Leaders:** You can use the book to prime yourself for any and all discussions of an environment of care nature with accreditation or facilities staff.

This Book Is for All Settings

You may be addressing air quality issues in a hospital surgical suite, suicide prevention in a community mental health center, hazmat spills in an ambulatory clinic, workplace violence in a nursing care center, or safe oxygen use in a patient's home. What you'll find as you read this book is that many Joint Commission standards related to the physical environment are mostly similar across the setting spectrum. And where there are major differences, this book will call them out for you.

This Book Focuses on the Basics

Whichever role you fill in whatever setting, you all need the same thing: a clear, easy-to-grasp guide to the environment of care basics. This book is it. What follows is an introduction to the basic concepts of the environment of care, which will be explained in this book.

Basic elements: The environment of care is made up of three basic elements that interact to create risk:

- **The physical space:** This includes the building structure, the required design interior elements, and the arrangement of the space.
- **The equipment and utilities:** This includes equipment and utilities that support patient care as well as the operation of the building.
- **The people:** This includes all who enter the environment—including patients, staff, vendors, and visitors. (In this book, contract workers and licensed independent practitioners are included in any mention of staff.)

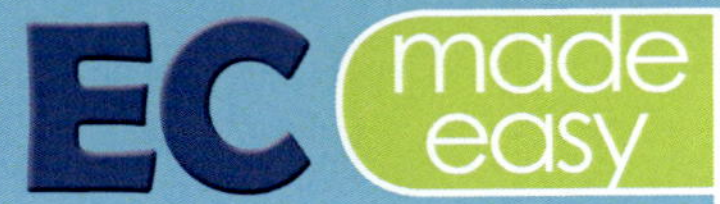

Basic risk areas and manual chapters: Joint Commission accreditation standards are designed to address risks. Standards related to risks in the physical environment appear in three chapters of the accreditation manual:

- **Environment of Care (EC):** The "Environment of Care" (EC) chapter covers what are known as the functional areas of the environment of care, as follows:
  - *Safety:* This area addresses risks usually related to accidental incidents that occur during everyday tasks, in the physical structure, or due to uncontrollable factors such as weather. It also includes worker safety and maintaining a healthy environment, one that is smoke-free, well-lit, and noise-controlled.
  - *Security:* This area addresses risks related to incidents that are often intentional and result in harm or loss to people and property (workplace violence, suicide, abductions, or theft). Access control is consequently a big part of security.
  - *Hazardous materials and waste:* To be compliant, you have to manage hazardous materials and waste from the time they enter the facility to the time they leave it. This area is all about managing the many risks involved in all the processes for handling these materials.
  - *Fire safety:* Fire protection is about preventing injury to life and/or property damage as a result of smoke, fire, and combustion. In the EC chapter, fire safety standards relate to efforts involving human intervention, such as fire drills and the testing and use of fire safety equipment.
  - *Medical equipment:* This area addresses risks related to equipment used in monitoring, treatment, diagnosis, or direct care of patients. Inventory, inspection, testing, and maintenance are primary activities involved in managing these risks.
  - *Utilities:* Risks in this area include (but aren't limited to) those related to electrical distribution, emergency power, vertical and horizontal transport, HVAC (heating, ventilating, and air-conditioning), plumbing, boiler and steam systems, piped medical gas, vacuum systems, and communication systems. Similar activities for managing medical equipment risks are applied in this area.

- **Emergency Management (EM):** Risks addressed in the standards of the "Emergency Management" (EM) chapter are related to any and all possible emergencies, including weather disasters, pandemics, or even terrorist situations. Activities revolve around mitigation, preparedness, response, and recovery.
- **Life Safety (LS):** Like fire safety, risks covered in the "Life Safety" (LS) chapter are about minimum requirements for systems and construction of a facility to offer protection from fire. In the LS chapter, fire safety standards relate to protection provided by building features and are written specifically to conform to the requirements of the *Life Safety Code®*.*

Book Organization and Format

You're busy, so this book is set up in a way that makes it easy to quickly find the information you need. Content is clearly labeled and consistently formatted, with core and extra features distinguished for targeted reading.

Parts of the book: The book is organized into three parts:
- **Part 1**
  - *Chapter 1:* Who's Who in EC
  - *Chapter 2:* What's What in EC
- **Part 2**
  - *Chapter 3:* Safety
  - *Chapter 4:* Security
  - *Chapter 5:* Hazardous Materials and Waste
  - *Chapter 6:* Medical Equipment and Utility Systems
  - *Chapter 7:* Fire Safety and Life Safety
  - *Chapter 8:* Emergency Management
  - *Chapter 9:* Construction
- **Part 3**
  - *Chapter 10:* The EC Survey

Chapter features: Each chapter includes the same types of features presented in the same order, so navigation is easy. And in the e-book version, internal links allow you to easily search for terms and navigate across chapters. Links even take you directly to the downloadable, customizable tools (in the print version, these tools are delivered on a flash drive).

* *Life Safety Code®* is a registered trademark of the National Fire Protection Association, Quincy, MA.

This chart shows the chapter features included in this book. Some features appear in the margins to correspond to the core content.

Chapter Feature	Purpose of Feature
The Big Idea	Presents the chapter theme/overview
Key Concepts	Highlights key ideas
In Other Words	Defines key terms in plain language
Collaboration	Explains how leaders, accreditation professionals, safety professionals, facilities directors, and other staff can work together
Smart Questions	Provides questions to begin focused conversation on environment of care subjects
From *EC News*	Offers related excerpts from *Environment of Care*® News
Picture THIS	Highlights topics visually
Tools of the Trade	Lists downloadable, customizable tools and how they can be used

A Note on the New Edition

The second edition of *EC Made Easy* has been updated to reflect a number of changes affecting environment of care and compliance issues, including the following:

- Total revision of The Joint Commission's Life Safety (LS) standards pursuant to the US Centers for Medicare & Medicaid Services' (CMS) adoption of the 2012 edition of the *Life Safety Code*
- Deletion and revision of several standards from The Joint Commission's Environment of Care (EC) standards
- Substantial revisions to The Joint Commission's accreditation process, including the methods used to assess a health care organization's level of compliance with the Survey Analysis for Evaluating Risk™ (SAFER™) matrix
- Changes to how The Joint Commission uses the Statement of Conditions™ (SOC) under the Life Safety standards

- Changes to The Joint Commission's post-survey process, including clarifications, time-limited waivers, equivalencies, interim life safety measures, plans for improvement, and survey-related plans for improvement

Acknowledgements

Joint Commission Resources gratefully acknowledges the time and insights of the subject matter experts at The Joint Commission. We would also like to thank our writer, James K. Foster.

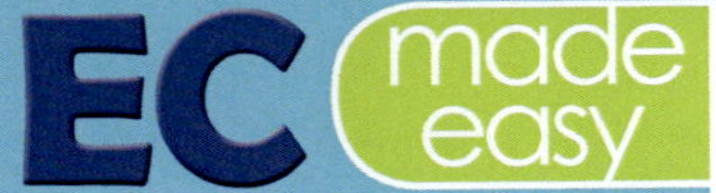

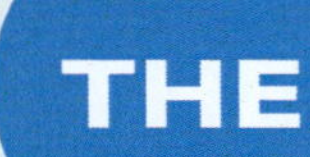

Who's Who in EC

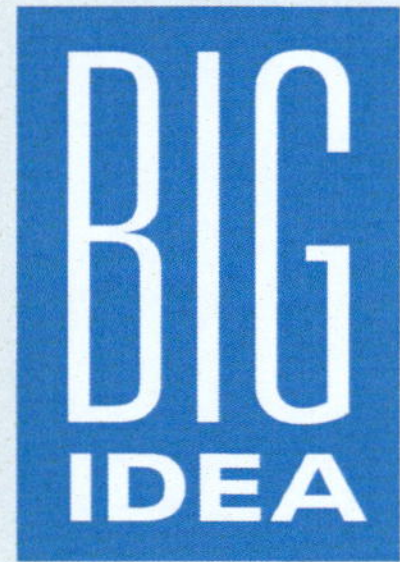

The environment of care field is both broad and deep. It involves everyone in the organization, not just the facilities team. That includes leaders and independent practitioners as well as clinical and environmental services staff. And everyone must understand and embrace this concept because how they act, how they react, and how they interact with everything and everyone in your organization can affect the safety of the environment of care. Getting to know all of the people and responsibilities involved in managing and maintaining the environment of care will help you create a successful team and a safe environment—whether you're overseeing the broad whole as a leader or accreditation professional, or are deep in the details as a facilities director.

KEY CONCEPTS

- [Responsibility for the Environment of Care](#)
- [Key Staff and Organizations](#)
- [The EC Committee](#)
- [Leadership Levels and PI](#)

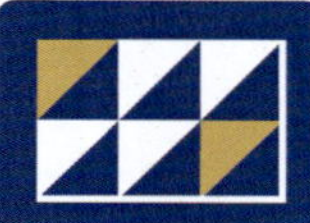

THE MANUAL

Following are the relevant Joint Commission *Comprehensive Accreditation Manual (CAM)* chapters:

- Environment of Care (EC)
- Human Resources (HR)
- Leadership (LD)
- Performance Improvement (PI)

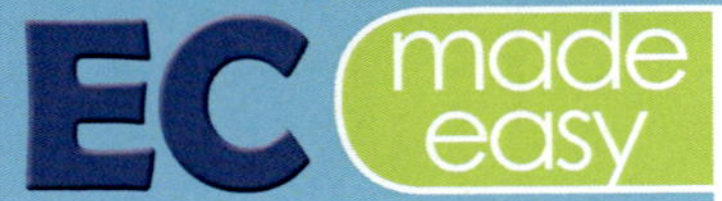

in other words

environment of care

The physical environment of a health care organization, which includes the building itself and its grounds, utilities, medical equipment, and more. Some organizations refer to this as the EOC, but that's not an acronym The Joint Commission uses.

risk

The probability that a disease, injury, condition, death, or related occurrence may occur for a person or population or that serious damage could occur to necessary equipment, the building, or property.

safety officer

A person who manages environmental risks and who also may be the person with authority to intervene when situations threaten people or property.

authority to intervene

A responsibility given to one or more individuals to step in and address environmental situations that can create immediate threats. This responsibility may be given to the same person who manages environmental risks.

Responsibility for the Environment of Care

Leaders are ultimately responsible for everything that happens in an organization, including anything in the environment of care. And accreditation professionals are indirectly responsible because they have to make sure the organization meets all the Joint Commission standards. But someone needs to be *directly* responsible for the environment of care. The Joint Commission requires your leaders (usually the CEO) to name one or more individuals to do just that. The individual(s) named fulfills two primary functions: managing environment of care risks and intervening in situations that pose an immediate threat to people or property. These functions can be assigned through job descriptions or in organization policies and procedures.

Environment of Care Risk Responsibility

Managing environment of care risks involves these three C's:
- **C**ollecting information about environment of care issues
- **C**onducting risk management activities
- **C**ommunicating the results of these activities

The safety officer: In many organizations, the risk responsibility function is performed by a safety officer. Large organizations may have a dedicated safety officer; small organizations might add this function to an existing environment of care- or accreditation-related position. Others might divide the responsibilities among several people—making clear roles and frequent communication extra important.

Authority to Intervene

Environmental situations can create immediate threats—to life and health, and to buildings, equipment, and property. These threats include such things as an unsafe work condition, hazardous materials spills, or security breaches. Authority to intervene in such situations is sometimes (but not always) assigned to the same person who manages environment of care risk.

Backup authority: You never know when a threat may emerge. So it's critical that someone with the authority to intervene is present in the organization at all times. But no single person can be on hand 24/7. That's why your organization needs to grant the authority to intervene to more than one person.

KEY CONCEPT

Key Staff and Organizations

The overarching environment of care label is applied to several broad and diverse subareas, addressed in the "Environment of Care" (EC) chapter of the accreditation manual: safety, security, hazardous materials and waste, fire safety, medical equipment, and utilities (*see* Chapters 3–7). Life safety (LS) and emergency management (EM) often carry the environment of care tag too (*see* Chapter 7 and Chapter 8, respectively). The safety officer (*see* above) could cover the entire lot; but in most organizations, various key staff hold positions of responsibility for the various subareas.

Key Staff

In the environment of care arena, you could interact with any one of the key staff named below (although they might have different titles). Most positions aren't explicitly required under Joint Commission standards, but each person fulfills an important role in maintaining environment of care safety.

- **Safety officer:** Identifies and manages risks related to the physical environment

- **Facilities director:** Manages the property or building, including operation, maintenance, and improvements

- **Vice president of construction/facilities/support services:** Plans and oversees construction or renovation projects

- **Emergency manager:** Acts as a contact or liaison between the EM team and other committees, such as the EC committee

- **Quality manager:** Manages emergency responses, such as using available resources. This role might be filled by the facilities director or another individual.

TRY THIS TOOL

Environment of Care Contact Sheet

You can use this form to collect contact information for environment of care staff and related staff you need to know in your organization.

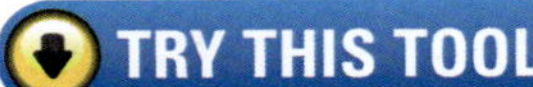

Security director: Protects people, property, and information, and responds to security incidents in the facility

Infection prevention and control practitioner: Oversees the organization's policies and procedures regarding infection, including how infection is affected by the physical environment

Radiation safety officer: Maintains safety in the use of radiation (in the radiology department)

Clinical engineer: Manages the implementation and use of medical equipment

Environmental services (EVS) director: Manages housekeeping, linen distribution, and waste management

Other contacts: You also want to get to know the go-to folks in areas that interact with the environment of care regularly, such as the laboratory and pharmacy, as well as the respiratory, nursing, materials management, and central sterile processing departments. Oh, and don't forget to connect with those in charge of your organization's overall risk management, accreditation and regulatory compliance, and performance improvement (PI) (*see* the Key Concept "Leadership Levels and PI" on page 9) activities.

COLLABORATION: Accreditation professionals, facilities directors, and leaders, be mindful that collaboration between clinical areas and environment of care areas is vital. For this reason, clinical representatives should be courted to work with key environment of care staff and consulted frequently on environment of care practices. It's also vital to collaborate with anyone in charge of meeting other requirements from local, state, and federal regulatory bodies.

Key Regulatory Organizations

The Joint Commission isn't the only organization with standards that impact environment of care activities in health care organizations. Here are some key national organizations you should know about:

in other words

performance improvement (PI)

The systematic process of identifying performance problems, developing and implementing solutions through interventions (actions), determining their success, and sustaining the improvement.

CDC and NIOSH: The Centers for Disease Control and Prevention (CDC) is an operating unit of the US Department of Health and Human Services. The CDC conducts research and investigations, and works to prevent and control the spread of infectious and contagious disease. The agency provides a surveillance system to monitor potential outbreaks and bioterrorism on a national and international basis. It's also involved with the prevention and control of injuries, workplace hazards, disabilities, and environmental health threats. The National Institute for Occupational Safety and Health (NIOSH) is part of the CDC and is responsible for research, education, information, and training in the field of occupational safety and health. You should be aware of CDC and NIOSH guidelines and helpful educational materials in relation to infection risks in the environment of care (*see* Chapter 3 and Chapter 5).

CMS: Accreditation from The Joint Commission can be used to meet certification standards for the US Centers for Medicare & Medicaid Services (CMS). It's known as deemed status, or deeming. This is possible because the standards and elements of performance (EPs) required for Joint Commission accreditation meet or exceed the standards set by CMS. CMS requirements are most often referred to as Conditions of Participation (CoPs) or Conditions for Coverage (CfCs).

- **Not for everyone:** Some standards listed in the *Comprehensive Accreditation Manuals* are required only for organizations seeking to use Joint Commission accreditation for deemed status purposes. These are always clearly marked in the standards, in **boldface.**
- **No guarantees:** Complying with Joint Commission standards and EPs will qualify your organization for CMS certification. However, be aware that compliance with CMS CoPs doesn't guarantee compliance with Joint Commission accreditation standards. Why not? Because some Joint Commission standards don't directly link to CoPs.

DOE: The US Department of Energy (DOE) advances the national, economic, and energy security of the United States; promotes scientific and technological innovation; and ensures environmental cleanup of the national nuclear weapons complex.

deemed status, deeming
Approval given by the US Centers for Medicare & Medicaid Services (CMS) to an organization like The Joint Commission that uses standards and survey processes equivalent to those used by Medicare or other federal programs to "deem" a health care organization as meeting such requirements. Those accredited organizations do not then have to go through the CMS survey and certification process; they are said to have "deemed status." Seeking deemed status through accreditation is an option, not a requirement. Deemed status is available for Joint Commission–accredited ambulatory surgical centers, clinical laboratories, critical access hospitals, home health agencies, hospice organizations, hospitals, and psychiatric hospitals.

From a health care perspective, the agency is concerned with radiation safety (*see* Chapter 5).

DOT: The US Department of Transportation (DOT) provides for the safety, adequacy, and efficiency of the transportation system, and included in this task is the safety of the transporation of hazardous materials (*see* Chapter 5).

EPA: The US Environmental Protection Agency (EPA) serves to protect human health and the environment, including developing and enforcing regulations related to hazardous materials (*see* Chapter 5).

FDA: The US Food and Drug Administration (FDA) ensures the safety of food, cosmetics, drugs for humans (and animals), the blood supply, and medical devices and equipment. The FDA also has enforcement authority, including product recalls, product seizures, and prosecution, so you might get notices from the FDA on product recalls (*see* Chapter 3).

FEMA: In addition to encouraging national emergency preparedness, the Federal Emergency Management Agency (FEMA) manages federal response and recovery efforts to any national emergency event. FEMA is part of the US Department of Homeland Security. You may have dealings with FEMA in relation to emergency management (*see* Chapter 8).

FGI: The Facility Guidelines Institute (FGI) is a private organization formed to provide for the ongoing review and revision of the *Guidelines for Design and Construction of Hospitals and Outpatient Facilities*. The 2014 edition is referenced by The Joint Commission (*see* Chapter 9).

NFPA: The National Fire Protection Association (NFPA) issues a code that specifies construction and operational conditions to minimize fire hazards and provide a system of safety in case of fire. The Joint Commission requires health care organizations to comply with this code, known as the *Life Safety Code*®,* as well as other codes from NFPA. To help assess compliance with the *Life Safety Code*, The Joint Commission created the "Life Safety" (LS) chapter, which includes all the Joint Commission requirements regarding *Life Safety Code* compliance. NFPA

* *Life Safety Code*® is a registered trademark of the National Fire Protection Association, Quincy, MA.

standards are also referenced in the EC standards in relation to fire safety (*see* Chapter 7).

NRC: The Nuclear Regulatory Commission (NRC) is an independent agency of the federal government charged with the regulation of nuclear materials by civilians (*see* Chapter 5).

OSHA: The Occupational Safety and Health Administration (OSHA) is a federal agency that aims to ensure employee safety and health in the United States by working with employers and employees to create better working environments. Its mission is to prevent work-related injuries, illnesses, and deaths. OSHA has a series of regulations that organizations must follow to ensure employee safety and health. You'll see references to OSHA throughout this book.

KEY CONCEPT

The EC Committee

Maybe the environment of care in your organization is managed single-handedly by the facilities director or safety officer. Or maybe it's the focus of a few professionals. Maybe there's a whole team of key staff working in tandem. In any case, most organizations also have an EC committee (sometimes called a safety committee) to help sort things out and get things done. It isn't required under Joint Commission EC standards, but it's considered a best practice.

EC Committee Duties

One of the most important typical duties of an EC committee is helping to create EC management plans (*see* Chapter 2). These plans include a process for monitoring and maintaining the environment of care, as required by Joint Commission standards.

Monitoring environment of care incidents: It's usually the EC committee members who monitor, investigate, and report internally on the following environment of care–related incidents when they occur:
- Security incidents
- Patient and guest injuries

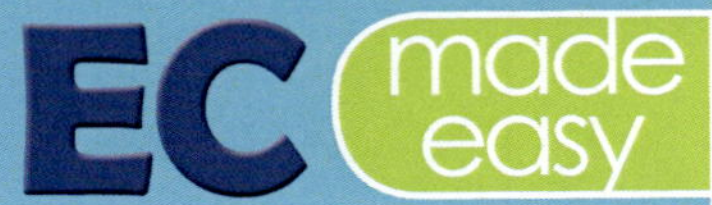

- Staff injuries and illness
- Hazardous materials spills and exposures
- Damage to property owned by the organization or others
- Recalls, alerts, and so on
- Problems, failures, or use errors in these areas:
  - Fire safety
  - Medical or laboratory equipment
  - Utilities

EC Committee Membership

Members of the EC committee are generally the same as the key EC staff (*see* page 3). Also crucial to include is the accreditation professional. And make sure that whoever is involved in creating management plans is on the committee because that's one of the common duties of committee members.

EC Committee Structure

Organizations structure EC committees in different ways. Following are three possible approaches to that structure. Of course, no matter how you structure it, the EC committee should report up the organizational quality and safety ladder, and ultimately be accountable to the leaders and the governing board.

The traditional approach: Basically, this is one committee, with members representing different EC subareas and related areas. It works best in small organizations; in large organizations, the committee may be so big that it's hard for all voices to be heard.

The subcommittee approach: This involves multiple subcommittees working independently on different EC subareas, reporting to a central EC steering committee. As long as the steering committee holds the subcommittees accountable, this system can be efficient and effective. See the sidebar "EC Subcommittees" for a list of possible EC subcommittees and their members.

The hybrid approach: A third option is a hybrid of the other two. Some of the subareas—for example, utilities and medical equipment—may be combined in a single standing committee working on its own but per the relevant management plan(s).

EC Subcommittees

Following is a list of possible subcommittees that might make up an EC committee. Some individuals or departments are repeated to show that they may provide input on multiple subcommittees. This is not an all-inclusive list; your organization should add or delete members as appropriate.

Safety Committee
Safety Officer
Public Safety
Guest Services
Employee Health
Nursing
Risk Management
Infection Control
Quality
Materials Management

Security Committee
Public Safety
Behavioral Health
Nursing
Guest Services
Facilities Engineering
Telecom
Emergency Department
Information Technology Security

Hazardous Materials Committee
Laboratory
Pharmacy
Nursing
Radiology
Environmental Services
General Supplies
Receiving and Supply Chain
Sterile Processing
Facilities Engineering
Emergency Department

Equipment Management Committee
Biomedical/Clinical Engineering
Nursing
Radiology
Anesthesia
Cardiology
Materials Management
Contract Management/Purchasing

Fire Prevention Committee
Public Safety
Facilities Engineering
Nursing
Guest Services
Laboratory

Utilities Management Committee
Facilities Engineering
Telecom
Information Systems
Respiratory
Nursing
Satellite Clinics

Education Committee
Human Resources
Nursing
Medical Staff
Public Relations
Marketing

Other Committees

Some functions of the EC committee will overlap or relate to those of other committees in your organization. These may include an EM committee, a fire safety committee, a patient safety committee, an infection control committee, and so on. Members of these committees will be valuable resources and may even participate in EC committee meetings and activities.

KEY CONCEPT

Leadership Levels and PI

As noted earlier, leaders are ultimately responsible for everything that happens in an organization. One of the most important aspects of their work is their role in PI efforts. The following is a summary of leaders at different levels and their responsibilities in that area.

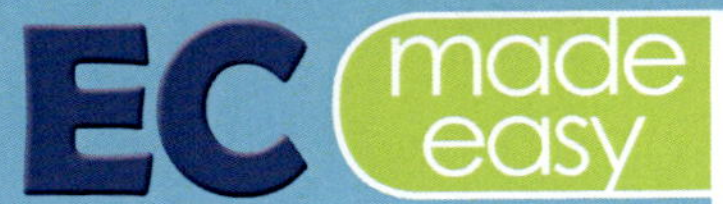

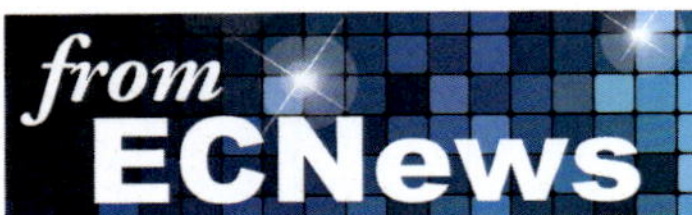

Coffee with the Crew

At 4:00 one afternoon your phone rings. It's the CEO, asking if he can come down to the power plant tomorrow at 7:30 a.m. and have coffee with you and your team. You respond enthusiastically, knowing this will give you an informal opportunity to communicate with a senior leader and help him see firsthand the daily challenges your department faces. This is not your first coffee meeting with the CEO. These meetings began a few months ago, and the success of the first interactions has led to regular "coffee with the crew" meetings . . . .

"For this interaction to be successful, both senior leaders and facilities staff will want to keep the tone informal and informative," says George Mills, Director of the Department of Engineering at The Joint Commission. "This is not the time to lecture or present a laundry list of complaints to leadership. The meeting should strictly focus on generating awareness and sharing information with leaders in a nonconfrontational way." . . . Ultimately, "coffee with the crew" can help organizations enhance communication between leadership and facility managers and build goodwill.

—excerpted from "Coffee with the Crew: Bringing Together Senior Leadership and Facility Management Staff to Discuss Facility Needs," *Environment of Care® News,* December 2011

Executive Leadership Level

- **Who they are:** Typically, this includes the board of directors (BOD), as well as the chief executive officer (CEO), chief operating officer (COO), chief medical officer (CMO), and chief nursing officer (CNO).
- **What they do:**
  - Set strategic imperatives
  - Provide resources
  - Heighten awareness of PI needs throughout the organization

Senior Leadership Level

- **Who they are:** Examples of individuals at this level include department chairs, medical and nursing directors, facilities directors, and accreditation and regulation professionals.
- **What they do:**
  - Coordinate the strategic imperatives set at the executive level
  - Analyze the current capacity to lead and spread PI
  - Define how to reach the goals and delegate resources
  - Monitor, respond to, and share PI reports

Frontline Leadership Level

- **Who they are:** This group may include attending physicians, clinical nurse specialists and other clinical leaders, staff nurses, patient care managers, and pharmacists.
- **What they do:**
  - Decide how to integrate PI interventions into clinical practice
  - Monitor effects of interventions
  - Evaluate the functionality of interventions
  - Provide education and rapid feedback on interventions to frontline staff
  - Make reports about interventions at regular meetings

TOOLS OF THE TRADE

- Environment of Care Contact Sheet
- Sample EC Committee Reporting Items Schedule

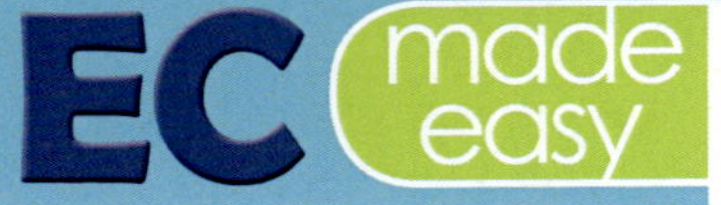

What's What in EC

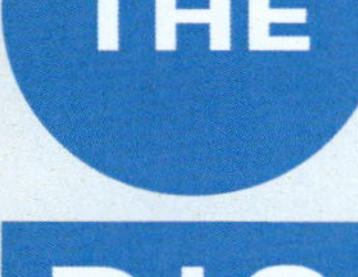
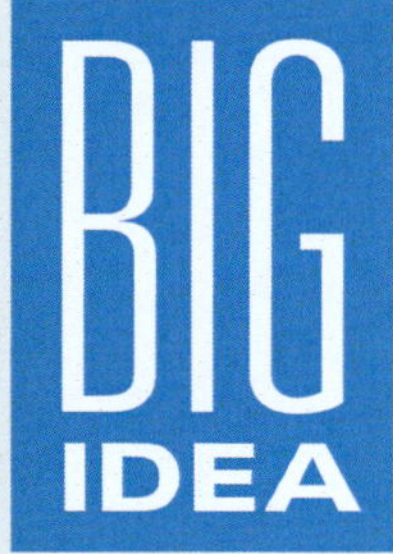

Managing the environment of care is complicated, but the job can be boiled down to a few basic, overarching tasks: defining strategies, responding to risks, and monitoring situations. Joint Commission requirements address those tasks as well as the strategies and tools needed to perform them: developing management plans, performing risk assessments, conducting environmental tours, and monitoring and making improvements. Accreditation professionals, leaders, and facilities directors or safety officers must work together, using these strategies and tools, to help an organization effectively manage the physical environment.

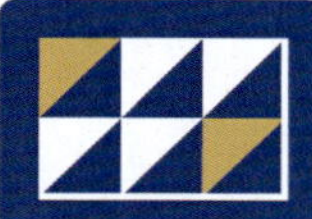

THE MANUAL

Following are the relevant Joint Commission *Comprehensive Accreditation Manual* (*CAM*) chapters:

- Environment of Care (EC)
- Human Resources (HR)
- Performance Improvement (PI)
- Leadership (LD)

KEY CONCEPTS

- EC Management Plans
- EC Risk Assessments
- Environmental Tours
- EC Documentation
- Improvement and ICES
- Competent, Well-Trained Facilities Staff

in other words

EC management plans
One or more written plans that provide an overview of an organization's approach to the environment of care and how that approach complies with Joint Commission Environment of Care (EC) standards.

smart questions:

What are the objectives of your organization's EC management plans?

EC Management Plans

Environment of Care (EC) standards compliance is too complex to navigate without road maps. That's where EC management plans come into play. These can be thought of as high-level business plans or executive summaries. They're a framework for management in relation to EC standards; they're *not* detailed descriptions of policies or procedures. You need these plans, which is why Joint Commission EC standards require them.

Purpose of EC Management Plans

Purpose drives process (and progress) in any endeavor. EC management plans have a dual purpose:

- To provide a framework for your organization's approach to the environment of care
- To briefly explain how that approach complies with Joint Commission EC standards

Other purposes: In addition, your management plans are extremely useful in the following ways:

- To help identify and manage risks
- To guide performance improvement (PI) efforts
- To provide leaders with a high-level view of environment of care activities
- To serve as a reference during tracers and on-site surveys
- To serve as an orientation document for new environment of care staff
- To guide ongoing environment of care education and training programs

Fundamentals of EC Management Plans

If your organization is accredited, you should already have management plans (though they might need improvement, of course). If you're applying for accreditation, you need to develop the plans. In any case, below are the fundamentals of EC management plans. (Also *see* the sidebars "Steps to Creating EC Management Plans" and "Do's and Don'ts of Creating EC Management Plans" on pages 17 and 18.)

Covering the EC areas: The Joint Commission requires management plans for the following functional areas, which are covered by the EC chapter in the accreditation manual:

- Safety
- Security
- Life safety
- Hazardous materials and waste (not required for behavioral health care organizations)
- Medical equipment management (not required for home care organizations; laboratory refers to this as laboratory equipment)
- Utility management

You can have a separate document for each of the EC functional areas, or you can combine them into one or more documents—whichever works best for your organization. An organization must also have a written Emergency Operations Plan (*see* Chapter 8) and a current Statement of Conditions™ (*see* Chapter 7). These are technically not management plans and have different parameters; however, they're integrally related to the EC standards.

Written documents: Per the standards, your management plans must be written. These are the documents that surveyors will reference and ask you about during survey, so they also need to be clearly written and easy to find. It's a good idea to have them labeled by version as well; that way, you know you're looking at the most current one.

Management plan elements: Each management plan, regardless of its EC area focus, should include the following common elements, and may also include a mission statement and other features:

- **Objectives:** Broad-based statements that discuss the purpose of the plan and what your organization hopes to accomplish in this EC area
- **Scope:** List or description of all your organization's sites covered by the plan (may also include hours of operation as well as services offered)

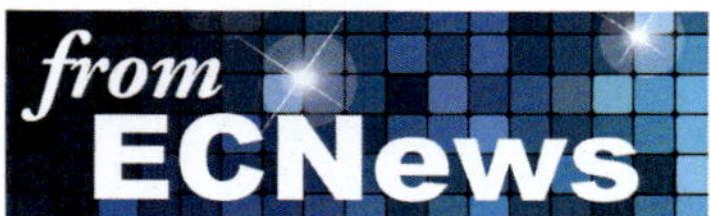

Consistent Structure

To ensure that your management plans are easy to navigate, understand, and use, you may want to keep the structure of the plans consistent.

For example, each plan could start with a mission and vision statement, a description of plan scope, and a list of objectives. A plan could then list compliance details and end with a brief discussion about how performance will be measured and how the plan will be evaluated. By keeping plans consistent, any individual can pick up any plan and know where to find certain information.

—excerpted from "Environment of Care Management Plans: Making sure your plans get the job done," by George Mills, Director of the Department of Engineering at The Joint Commission, *Environment of Care® News*, June 2013

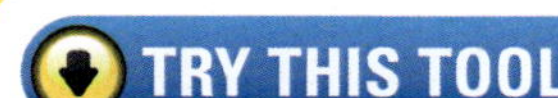

Sample Safety Management Plan

You can use this sample safety management plan as a template for your own EC management plans or compare it to your existing plans and look for ways to improve them.

- **Performance:** Description of how your organization will measure the performance of the plan in reducing risk and keeping patients, visitors, and staff safe
- **EP compliance:** Brief description of how each element of performance (EP) for each EC standard in the EC area will be met (keeping in mind that surveyors will hold you accountable for what your policies state you'll do to maintain compliance, so be realistic)
- **Responsibilities:** Information on general and/or specific responsibilities of individuals and groups for compliance and other activities
- **Time frames:** Notations regarding time frames for performing specific compliance activities
- **Emergency response:** Summary of how to respond to particular emergency situations, further described in the Emergency Operations Plan (*see* Chapter 8)
- **Inspection, testing, and maintenance:** Description of your approach to these activities, per the respective standards
- **Policies and procedures:** Citations or cross-references to your organization's relevant policies and procedures
- **Supplemental information:** References to critical related information, such as municipal codes
- **Risk assessment:** Explanation of how risk assessments will be used in risk management of the EC area
- **Staff development:** Explanation of how staff (including contract staff) will be oriented and trained
- **Annual evaluation:** Description of how annual evaluation of the plan will be conducted and by whom

Related EPs from non-EC chapters: EC management plans need to be comprehensive. So they should also address standards and EPs in other chapters of the accreditation manual related to the environment of care. Make sure your plans incorporate cross-referenced EPs in the following manual chapters, especially the first two:

- Life Safety (LS)
- Emergency Management (EM)
- Human Resources (HR)
- Infection Prevention and Control (IC)
- Information Management (IM)
- Leadership (LD)
- Performance Improvement (PI)

Multidisciplinary approach: Your management plans must take into consideration the various departments and staff they directly affect. Make sure to include feedback from these individuals when developing and reviewing your management plans.

Authority having jurisdiction (AHJ): Your management plans must be compliant with the strictest authority having jurisdiction (AHJ). Always follow the most stringent regulations that apply to your organization—even if they are "just" local. Any variation from Joint Commission standards should be highlighted in your management plan to clarify that for surveyors.

in other words

authority having jurisdiction (AHJ)
The organization, office, or individual responsible for approving equipment, materials, an installation, or a procedure.

Steps to Creating EC Management Plans

➤ **Step 1 — Determine the focus:** Decide whether to create individual or consolidated plans for the functional EC areas.

➤ **Step 2 — Choose a format:** Review other organizations' plans or canned plans to get ideas. Consider how to include elements needed in the annual evaluation, such as objectives, scope, performance, and evaluation.

➤ **Step 3 — Create an outline:** This should be based on the EC standards and elements of performance (EPs). Each EP must be addressed.

➤ **Step 4 — Address related regulations:** Add issues related to the following:
  – Stricter and strictest requirements of other agencies
  – Unlisted regulatory issues
  – Other related Joint Commission standards

➤ **Step 5 — Describe compliance:** Briefly explain compliance with each EP.

➤ **Step 6 — Identify responsibilities:** Identify the responsibilities of individuals or groups, especially those related to compliance activities.

➤ **Step 7 — Include time frames:** Specify time frames, per the standards, for completing required compliance tasks.

➤ **Step 8 — Cross-reference other documents:** Add references to more detailed organization policies and procedures as well as any relevant supplemental information.

➤ **Step 9 — Address monitoring performance:** Identify appropriate performance monitors, based on actual or potential risk.

➤ **Step 10 — Define data processes:** Establish and document the process of information collection and evaluation, including that for performance improvement.

➤ **Step 11 — Incorporate training:** Determine the content and establish the process for staff orientation and education on EC issues.

➤ **Step 12 — Specify document review:** Establish the process for annual evaluation of the management plan.

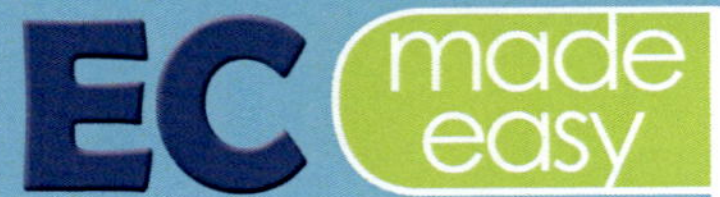

in other words

A review every 12 months of EC management plans to make sure the plans are still relevant, applicable, and effective, and reflect any changes at the organization.

> **TRY THIS TOOL**
>
> **EC Management Plan Evaluation Checklist**
> You can use this checklist to determine the quality and completeness of your EC management plans.

COLLABORATION: Creating management plans is an excellent opportunity for collaboration. Safety officers, facilities directors, and accreditation professionals, you may want to create the draft plans together, get review from subject matter experts (like hazardous waste disposal services), and then run the plans by leaders. In some cases, you may turn over the drafting of plans to EC–area leaders, such as the security director for the security plan. Leaders, you need to be ready to supply input and approval. This kind of team effort can build better-rounded plans—and foster beneficial buy-in.

Annual Evaluation of EC Management Plans

Things change. So your management plans may need to change too. Per the standards, EC management plans must undergo an annual evaluation (every 12 months) to make sure they're still relevant, applicable, and effective. Evaluating the plans doesn't necessarily mean they have to be changed. But your plans need to reflect the current situation and environment at your organization.

Do's and Don'ts of Creating EC Management Plans

Remember these tips when you're writing management plans:

✔ **DO** keep consistent structure in all management plans to make them easy to understand, navigate, and update.

✔ **DO** refer to relevant supporting policies or documentation.

✔ **DO** make sure each management plan reflects actual practice in the organization, including practices specific to certain sites.

✖ **DON'T** get too detailed on the "how" (these are not operational plans).

✖ **DON'T** simply restate the standards and elements of performance (EPs).

✖ **DON'T** treat management plans as just one more matter of compliance.

✖ **DON'T** just insert your organization's name into a set of canned plans.

Aspects to review: The annual evaluation should review the following aspects of the management plans, which is what surveyors will score them on, as well as a general review of the elements of the plans:

- **Objectives:** Does each objective still match the needs of the organization?
- **Scope:** Has anything changed in the organization's composition (facilities, hours of operation, services offered) that needs to be updated in the plans?
- **Performance:** Are the plans working? You might want to include as an addendum a summary of PI data collected during the year, and/or a record of mandatory compliance activities such as drills or maintenance.
- **Effectiveness:** Does the practice reflect the plans? What went well during the year? What could be improved?

Getting buy-in by getting input: When you evaluate the plans, be sure to involve the people who deal with the real-world implementation of those plans, such as frontline staff, nurses, and department heads. They can point out strengths and weaknesses in the plans. If possible, document exactly who suggested what, so you can go back to get feedback on implementation from the original sources of the suggestions. When contributors see the value of their input, they're more likely to continue to offer it.

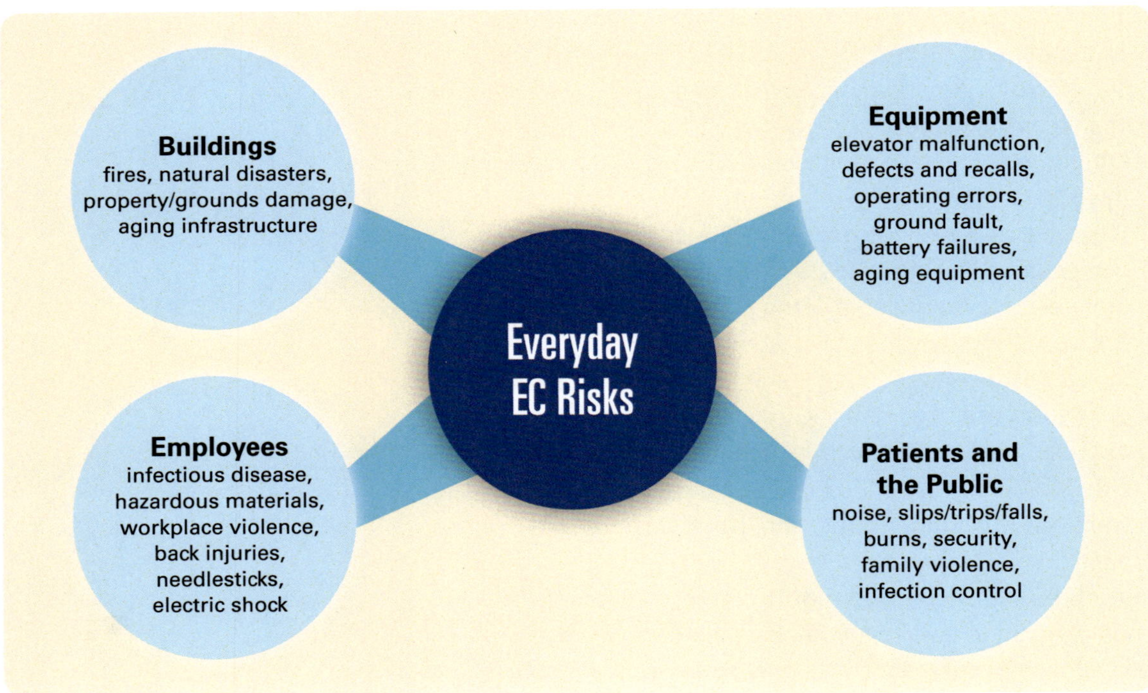

in other words

risk assessment

An examination of a function or process to determine the actual and potential risks and prioritize areas for improvement.

EC Risk Assessments

Risk is common in the physical environment—affecting buildings, equipment, employees, patients, and the public. Joint Commission EC standards require you to identify these risks using risk assessments and to make efforts to minimize or eliminate those risks. In fact, your risk management approach should be woven throughout your EC management plans (*see* above).

Purpose of EC Risk Assessment

You can meet the compliance goal for risk assessments by ensuring that they fulfill the following dual purpose:

- To identify potential risks to safety
- To determine what action, if any, is necessary to improve safety

Other purposes: Risk assessments also serve lots of other valuable purposes:

- To improve the safety of everyone in the physical environment—patients, staff, visitors
- To increase efficiency by forcing your organization to look at its processes objectively (rather than just doing things the same old way)
- To identify areas where more training is needed to avoid risk
- To serve as training tools to build awareness of risky situations
- To demonstrate to leadership the need for new equipment, staff, or space
- To facilitate collaboration in addressing a particular issue
- To help prioritize performance improvement initiatives

Identifying Risks in EC Areas

When it comes to risk management, you have to look at what's happening and what might happen. That's how to prevent harm and keep everyone safe—and that means *everyone*: patients, staff, visitors, vendors, contract workers, and so on.

Risks in the EC areas: Each of the functional areas of the EC has inherent risks, so your organization needs to identify risks and conduct risk assessments in each of those areas. In addition, construction or renovation requires its own separate risk assessment. Following is a brief description of the types of risks to look for in each EC area risk assessment (more detail on these will be in the related chapters of this book):

- **Safety:** Risks in safety address potential accidents, such as slips/trips/falls, as well as risks related to worker safety, controlling noise, and other environmental elements (*see* Chapter 3).
- **Security:** These types of risks are the results of intentional actions (theft, abduction, violence) and can be caused by individuals from inside or outside the organization. Your organization may want to do special planning to make sure the security needs of vulnerable populations (pediatric, geriatric, behavioral health) are covered (*see* Chapter 4).
- **Fire safety:** These risks are related to your organization's fire response, including drills that test performance of staff and fire safety equipment (*see* Chapter 7).

- **Hazardous materials and waste:** Risks in this area include all the processes involved in handling and disposing of dangerous materials, including risks during emergencies and accidental spills. Use of an inventory of hazardous materials is typically part of the risk assessment (*see* Chapter 5).
- **Medical equipment:** Risks in this area revolve around proper inspection, testing, and maintenance as well as use of new equipment. A medical equipment inventory is central to controlling these risks (*see* Chapter 6).
- **Utilities:** Risks in this area are like those in medical equipment but address electrical, water, medical gas, vacuum, heating, ventilation, and air-conditioning systems—and include potential failures of those systems. A utilities inventory is critical to managing these risks (*see* Chapter 6).
- **Preconstruction:** Proactive risk assessments must be conducted before a new construction or renovation project. They address the potential risks to existing occupied spaces caused by the work, such as compromised fire alarm systems or security of the construction areas (*see* Chapter 9).

High-risk locations and populations: It'll probably come as no surprise that some locations and patient populations are more prone to certain EC–area risks than others. Overall, these include, but aren't limited to, the following:

- **Buildings and grounds:** Security, safety, utilities
- **Emergency department:** Security (including violence), safety, medical equipment
- **Laboratory:** Security, hazardous materials and waste, fire safety
- **Pharmacy:** Security, hazardous materials and waste
- **Radiology:** Medical equipment, safety
- **Behavioral health:** Security (violence, including suicide)
- **Home care:** Security (in homes and neighborhoods)
- **Geriatric:** Safety, security (including elopement/wandering)
- **Pediatrics:** Security, safety
- **Women's health; mother and baby units:** Security
- **Operating and procedure rooms:** Security, utilities

Risk assessment sources: The Joint Commission requires organizations to use internal and external sources to identify areas for risk assessment. These may include the following:

- Internal performance improvement data

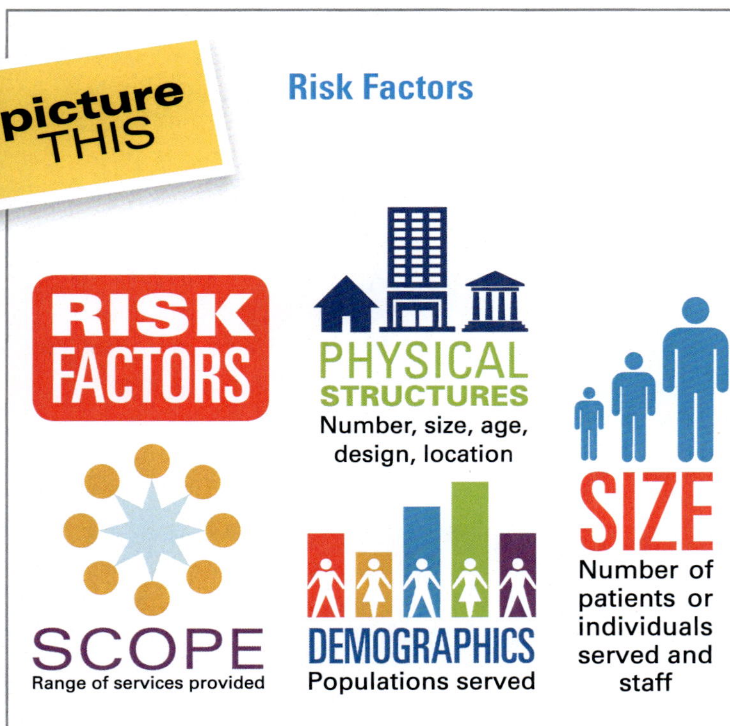

- Staff feedback
- Patient and family feedback
- Environmental monitoring activities
- Results of annual proactive risk assessments
- Results of any root cause analysis
- Data from sister, parent, or similar organizations on a local, state, or national level
- State or national professional organizations and associations
- National safety organizations, such as the ECRI Institute, the Institute for Healthcare Improvement, and the National Patient Safety Foundation
- Government agencies such as the Occupational Safety and Health Administration (OSHA)
- Association/society/professional literature
- *Sentinel Event Alert* and Sentinel Event Database
- Liability insurance company data

in other words

root cause analysis
One of several comprehensive systematic analysis methods for identifying the basic or causal factor(s) underlying variation in performance.

sentinel event
A patient safety event (not primarily related to the natural course of the patient's illness or underlying condition) that reaches a patient and results in death, permanent harm, or severe temporary harm. See the "Sentinel Event" (SE) chapter of the *Comprehensive Accreditation Manual* for a list of sentinel events, including those related to the environment of care.

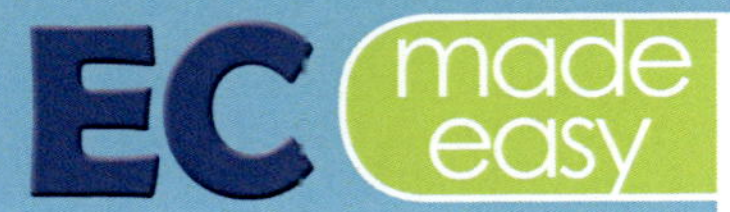

Relevant, specific risks: Targeting general EC–area risks and high-risk areas is a good starting point. But a risk assessment is most useful if it addresses a specific issue that's relevant to your organization.

COLLABORATION: Facilities directors, when you're identifying risks, reach out to get targeted perspectives on organization-specific issues to focus on. Accreditation professionals, you can work with the facilities director to point out some that are related to compliance issues. And leaders, remember that it's your responsibility to actually choose and approve any PI initiatives related to risk assessment results.

Performing Risk Assessments

No single prescribed format is required for conducting risk assessments. The risk factors (size, scope, demographics, and physical structures) of your organization will help shape what your risk assessments will look like.

Risk assessment process: If you use a standardized approach for risk assessments, the process may go more smoothly because everyone knows "what's next." The following approach can be used as a jumping-off point for creating your own approach—standardized or not:

Step 1 — Identify the issue: Keep it simple and specific. You might phrase your risk assessment objective as a statement ("Require visitors to wear identification badges in high-security areas.") or as a yes/no question ("Should we require visitors to wear identification badges in high-security areas?").

Step 2 — List advantages: Develop arguments for addressing the proposed issue by defining advantages— reasons that support doing so. Include evidence to support your reasons. Things to consider include the impact on patient care delivery, staff, the work environment, visitors, public safety, finances, and so on.

Step 3 — List disadvantages: Develop arguments against addressing the proposed issue by identifying concerns or risks associated with it. These should also be supported with evidence. Consider the same variables as in Step 2.

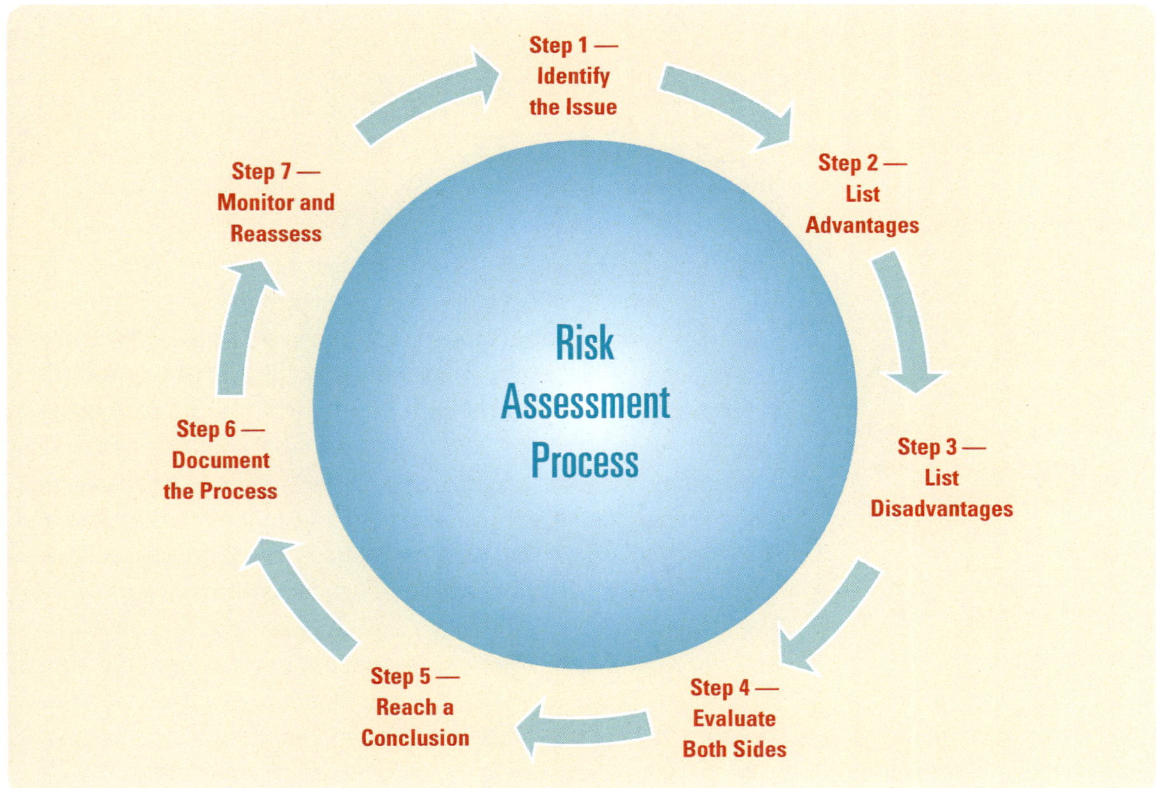

Step 4 — Evaluate both sides: Quantify the risk to the organization. Consider a scoring technique to determine if the risk is high, moderate, or low. Consider the probability of an adverse event occurring. Be impartial. Involve all the stakeholders who will be affected by the decision.

Step 5 — Reach a conclusion: Decide to either accept the risk or to take steps to minimize it. After deciding, you may want to share your report with the EC committee and patient safety committee to make sure there's consensus.

Step 6 — Document the process: Keep a written record of the whole risk assessment process. Update any relevant policies or procedures.

Step 7 — Monitor and reassess: Before any changes are implemented, define how the issue will be monitored up front (*see* the Key Concept "Improvement and ICES" on page 30). This should include a specific time frame to see if the interventions have had the results you wanted. If they have, document it and decide if you need more monitoring. If not, send the issue back through the risk assessment cycle.

smart questions:

During EC risk assessments, how often do you circle back to reassess the issue?

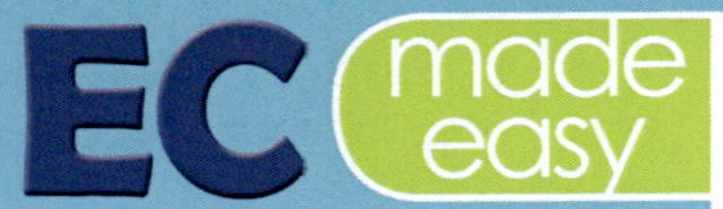

(For a real-world example of a risk assessment process, *see* the sidebar, "Sample Risk Assessment: Exposed Plumbing in a Behavioral Unit" on page 55.)

KEY CONCEPT

Environmental Tours

Although not required by Joint Commission standards, an environmental tour (EC tour) could be one of the most critical activities your organization performs. It can be an essential component of risk assessment (described above) as well as improvement (described below). Environmental tours can compliment the organization's Building Maintenance Program (BMP) as you search for items and objects that are subject to routine failure. Deficiencies identified in an environmental tour can be tracked and managed in a BMP with written strategies, documented schedules for inspections, and processes for evaluating effectiveness.

Not patient safety tours: Note that EC tours are not the same as patient safety tours. An EC tour is focused on the environmental factors affecting the safety and security of everyone in the facility; patient safety tours focus on clinical safety.

Performing EC Tours: Where, When, and Who

An EC tour isn't an ad hoc activity. It needs careful planning to be done correctly and effectively. The why is obvious, but you need to plan—and communicate the plan—regarding where, when, and who.

Where to perform EC tours: Areas toured should include any and all facility areas, not just those where patients receive care. Plan the EC tours to include public waiting areas, grounds, sidewalks, parking areas, doors, walkways, stairs (inside and outside), and elevators.

When to perform EC tours: Environmental tours should be based on the needs and reliability of maintaining a safe environment in both patient and non–patient care areas.

Who should perform EC tours: Ideally, the EC tour should be a multidisciplinary team effort. At the core of the team are the

in other words

environmental tour

A routine comprehensive facility tour to evaluate environmental conditions and the effectiveness of current practice in managing environmental safety risks. This tour is not required by the standards.

Building Maintenance Program (BMP)

A method for tracking, managing, and correcting deficiencies through maintenance activities. The program can consist of written strategies to manage items covered in the program, a documented schedule for the frequency of inspecting the items, and processes for evaluating the effectiveness of the program.

safety officer and the head of the department or unit in question. Staff of the department being toured should participate, as well as representatives from the following areas:

- Security
- Housekeeping/environmental services
- Infection control
- Nursing
- Medical staff
- Facility engineering
- Clinical engineering
- Pharmacy (if part of the organization)
- Administration

COLLABORATION: Accreditation professionals, it's a good idea for you to participate in these tours or receive documentation on them. Leaders, your representation is also encouraged. And safety officers or facilities directors, think about inviting individuals who have experience with specific patient populations, such as geriatric, pediatric, or psychiatric populations. They may notice potential EC risks that others might miss.

How to Perform EC Tours

To be effective, an EC tour needs to be more than just walking around and pointing out problems. How your organization conducts its EC tours likely will be unique. It's a best practice, however, to include several different information-gathering methods to get the full picture.

Visual observations: This is physically looking at the environment and the way things work in that environment. Here are some issues to pay attention to:

- **Hazards and safety issues:** The many and varied potential problems here include cluttered corridors, inadequate lighting, tripping hazards, and so on.
- **Proper storage:** Depending on your organization, you may need to consider how a whole range of items are stored, such as needles/sharps, supplies, food, medication, blood products, cleaning supplies, linens, hand hygiene products (alcohol gels, gloves, paper towels), and medical equipment.
- **Workarounds:** These are shortcuts that staff sometimes take to save time, such as disabling a door latch or leaving

In the last week, have you seen anything in your facility that should be fixed before the next EC tour?

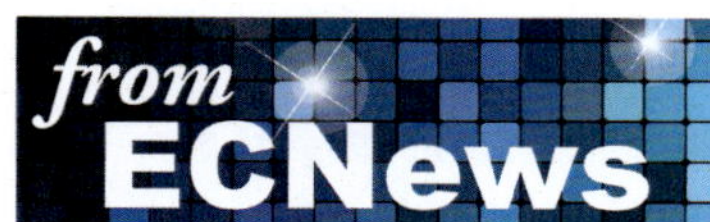

Safety Champions and EC Tours
Safety champions are people selected from each unit, department, or area who are specially trained to advocate safety and promote safety awareness in their work environment. Safety champions also disseminate appropriate education to the other members of their unit or department, as directed by the safety officer. . . .

[If] safety champions are included in the tours as observers and to help identify deficiencies, they will have a vested interest in making sure those deficiencies are corrected and in motivating their colleagues to maintain that safety. They can provide verification that items identified as potentially unsafe are corrected in a timely manner.

—excerpted from "Safety Champions: Making Health Care Safety Everyone's Business," by George Mills, Director of the Department of Engineering at The Joint Commission, *Environment of Care*® News, February 2013

security-sensitive supplies unattended while seeing to other tasks. (*See* Chapter 3 for more on workarounds.)

Staff interviews: Talking to people is a great way to find out what's *really* going on in the physical environment. And ad hoc interviews with staff members can shed light on their awareness of policies and procedures that relate to EC areas such as safety, security, fire safety, and medical equipment. This interactive approach can also serve as an educational opportunity to teach staff—and learn from them.

Pre-tour document review: Before touring a particular area or department, the EC tour team should consider going over any relevant written policies or procedures. With those fresh in mind, it'll be easier to recognize any discrepancies between policy and practice. Other documentation that might be reviewed as part of the tour is employee orientation and education and product recall notifications.

EC Tour Follow-Up

Your EC tour will be a waste of time if you don't do anything with the information gathered. Any problems identified should be addressed using a defined process of assessment, action, and reassessment. That process should be outlined in your EC management plans.

Immediate threats: If the EC tour team identifies an environmental issue that poses immediate threat to life, health, or safety, the problem should be corrected immediately and reported to the appropriate department manager. Accreditation professionals and the affected department staff should keep an eye on it to make sure it doesn't crop up again. Note: This isn't the same thing as *Immediate Threat to Life* (*ITL*), something identified by a surveyor during a survey. (*See* Chapter 10 for more information on ITLs.)

Less immediate threats: Other problems may require attention too, but not immediately. The EC tour team can create a follow-up report that outlines problems uncovered and opportunities for improvement, and then designate time frames for correcting each problem. This report can be given to depart-

⊙ TRY THIS TOOL

EC Tour Checklist
You can adapt this tool for your EC tour to make sure nothing gets overlooked. Consider assigning sections to EC tour team members.

ment leaders for action. After the designated time frame, another tour can be conducted to reassess—that is, see if the problem has been corrected.

Tour results: An overview of the EC tour findings can be shared with organization leadership and other groups, such as the patient safety and/or PI committee.

EC Rounds

Some organizations have incorporated a daily EC round into their risk management approach. Borrowing from the practice of clinicians, who visit their patients every day, environment of care facilities directors or safety officers visit key areas every day. They're not required by The Joint Commission, but EC rounds are a good way to keep on top of conditions in the physical environment. Similar to EC tours, EC rounds can be used as a monitoring tool to assess everyday risks and catch basic EC issues right away, before they become a hazard. Participating in EC rounds frequently can help accreditation professionals (and leaders) keep their finger on the pulse of EC safety and continuous compliance.

KEY CONCEPT

EC Documentation

A good rule of thumb in the EC world is, "Not documented, not done." You need documentation to manage maintenance, plan construction projects, keep track of monitoring data, and more.

Required Written Documentation

Documentation is performed for practical purposes and to help ensure a safe environment. Joint Commission surveyors want to see documentation of the EPs with required written documentation (RWD). These are identified in the accreditation manuals (and in the E-dition®, the electronic version of the manuals) with the Ⓓ icon. The Accredited Survey Activity Guide for Health Care Organizations, available on your *Joint Commission Connect™* extranet site, includes a handy addendum: the Life Safety and Environment of Care – Document List and Review Tool. (More on EC documentation in Chapter 10.)

⊙ TRY THIS TOOL

EC Assessment Checklist
Adapt this handy tool for your regular EC rounds.

---

in other words

EC round

A daily walkthrough of an area in which staff look for basic EC issues that can be corrected right away, rather than waiting until the more in-depth environmental tour. This type of monitoring is not required under Joint Commission standards.

---

in other words

required written documentation (RWD)

A procedure, policy, plan, license, or other piece of written information that goes beyond what is included in a medical record and is necessary for accreditation compliance. The documentation can be on paper or in an electronic format.

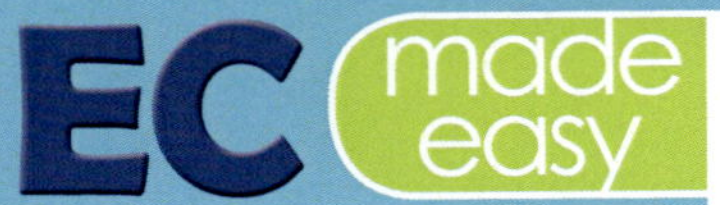

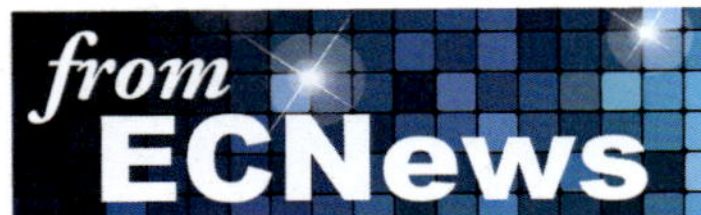

Contractor Documentation

A simple solution to managing documentation and associated actions related to the features of fire protection for work performed by outside contractors involves including in the request for bids a requirement that, at the end of each day, the contractor must provide a list of all discovered failed devices. [The contractor is still responsible for a complete and detailed list at the end of the project.] The organization can then use the list to correct the deficiencies. Once the inspection concludes, the organization will have records that all devices were tested and any that failed were corrected as soon as possible.

—adapted from "Comprehensive Documentation Demonstrates a Safe Environment: EC, EM, and LS Records Critical to Monitoring and Improving Performance," by George Mills, Director of the Department of Engineering at The Joint Commission, *Environment of Care®* News, November 2012

in other words

Information Collection and Evaluation System (ICES)

A structure for collecting and responding to information about deficiencies in the physical environment.

While the manuals should be your primary source to see which EPs require written documentation, here are a few that facility directors and accreditation professionals alike will want to keep in mind.

EC management plans documentation: As explained above, these written plans summarize how the organization is meeting EPs in each of the EC functional areas.

Fire response documentation: A written fire response plan is required. It describes the specific roles of staff and licensed independent practitioners at and away from a fire's point of origin, including when and how to sound and report fire alarms, how to contain smoke and fire, how to use a fire extinguisher, and how to evacuate to areas of refuge. The critiques of the drills and evaluation of the critiques must be documented too. Plus, inspection, testing, and maintenance, of all fire safety features needs to be documented (*see* Chapter 7).

Inventory documentation: Both medical equipment and utility components require written inventories in most organizations (check your manual). These must feature a list of items included in the inventory; a description of required inspection, testing, and maintenance activities; and how often those must be completed. You must also document the results of the inspection, testing, and maintenance. A written procedure must be in place to deal with clinical interventions in the case of utility or equipment failures. (For more on inventories, *see* Chapter 6.)

KEY CONCEPT

Improvement and ICES

No organization is perfect. Incidents and deficiencies happen. The important thing is to deal with them effectively. To do this, you have to continuously measure, assess, and improve. The way your organization does this in the physical environment is known as your Information Collection and Evaluation System (ICES). This concept appears in Joint Commission Standard EC.04.01.01.

Collecting ICES Data

To measure performance, you must first collect data, of course. And that takes a coordinated effort. Your organization should collect data about environment of care issues and incidents that occur across the entirety of your organization. That's how you can tell if something is a problem in one location or all locations, in one EC area or in all EC areas.

Data in ICES: Here are some examples of data your ICES should include, broken down by EC area:
- **Safety:** Incidents of property damage, patient and visitor injury, occupational illness, and worker safety injuries or issues
- **Security:** Security incidents involving patients, visitors, personnel, or property
- **Hazardous materials and waste:** Spills and exposures
- **Fire safety:** Deficiencies and failures in protecting occupants
- **Medical equipment:** Medical equipment failures, user errors, Safe Medical Devices Act issues, or product recalls
- **Utilities:** Utility failures and environmental issues, including proper temperature and humidity levels

Sources of risk data: You should also gather data about situations that could lead to future incidents—risk assessment data. And be sure the data you collect indicate actual risks and are meaningful. Include details that demonstrate why the situation is a risk. In addition to the risk assessment data sources listed above, these data can be collected from several sources:
- Environmental rounds or tours (if conducted)
- Staff assessments
- Satisfaction surveys from patients and staff
- Product recalls and alerts
- Regulatory updates

Performance monitoring: Data collection is part of performance monitoring, which is required by the standards. In addition to collecting data on incidents and risks, that monitoring should also include looking for processes that can be improved and provide opportunities to trend for improvement.

Your organization may already use specific types of performance monitors, so consulting with your PI team is a good first step to incorporating those into your ICES.

Sorting and Using ICES Data

When you have the raw data, you need to organize the information in a way that makes sense of it and renders it usable. Some organizations use spreadsheets, others dashboards. You may want to sort the data according to the functional EC areas. Putting data related to each area into separate documents helps relevant data flow to the proper channels (the EC committee, for example).

From information to improvement: When you put the data into a usable form, the information can be analyzed—and a response can be designed. Issues may be identified as opportunities for improvement and prioritized. Specific issues may be selected as PI projects. Keep this in mind: EC standards require an organization to undertake *at least one* environment of care PI project *every* year. Leaders, in particular, because they're charged with selecting and approving PI projects, should be very interested in ICES data.

Competent, Well-Trained Facilities Staff

Every organization knows the value of hiring competent, well-trained staff. But even if you hire competent and well-trained staff, you have to keep them competent and well-trained. Plus, you have to orient them to the particulars of your organization. The Joint Commission has orientation, education, and training requirements in almost every chapter of the accreditation manual, including those for EC, EM, and LS standards.

Education on Environment of Care Topics

One of the reasons this book exists is because the environment of care is a difficult and broad-ranging topic with lots of technical details and nuances. It isn't easy to learn or teach. Facilities

---

staff, like staff in other areas of your organization, are going to need education on environment of care issues. And it isn't just facilities staff who need environment of care education—it's everyone in your organization.

Specific topics: Here are environment-related topics that everyone will need to know about, in addition to orientation and competency assessments for job responsibilities:

- How to report concerns about environmental safety in your organization
- Roles and responsibilities in fire drills
- How to identify environment of care risks
- How to respond to environment of care incidents
- Communication of information and instructions in emergencies
- Roles and responsibilities during an emergency
- Safety content
- Responsibilities related to preventing and controlling infections
- Building deficiencies, construction hazards, and temporary measures taken to maintain fire safety and life safety
- Purpose and correct operation of alarm systems

TOOLS OF THE TRADE

- Sample Safety Management Plan
- EC Management Plan Evaluation Checklist
- EC Tour Checklist
- EC Assessment Checklist
- Mock Tracer Worksheet with SAFER™ Matrix: EC Performance Monitoring

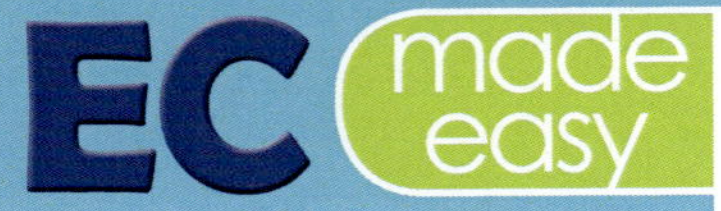

Chapter 3
Safety

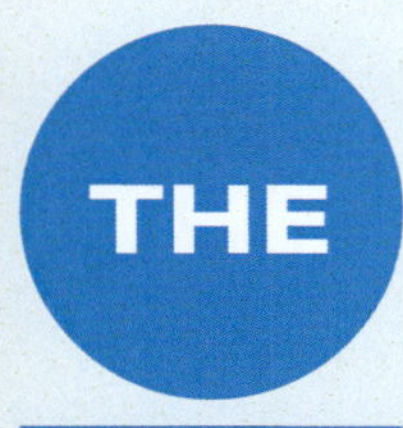

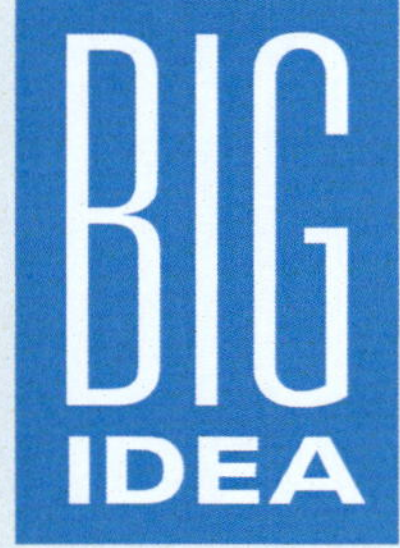

It's better to be safe than sorry—especially in health care organizations, where staff, patients, and visitors interact in an environment rife with potential hazards. The Joint Commission requires your organization to effectively manage safety risks addressed by Environment of Care (EC) safety standards, which are generally related to *accidental* incidents. This requires a solid understanding of safety issues such as safe workplace practice, ergonomics, infection control, slips/trips/falls hazards, and well-marked equipment. It also requires understanding factors related to maintaining a healthy environment, such as prohibiting smoking, ensuring adequate lighting, and maintaining clean facilities.

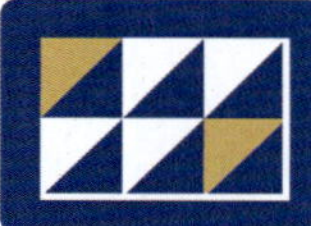

THE MANUAL

Following are the relevant Joint Commission *Comprehensive Accreditation Manual* (*CAM*) chapters:

- Environment of Care (EC)
- Infection Prevention and Control (IC)
- Leadership (LD)

KEY CONCEPTS

- General Safety
- Worker Safety
- Infection in the Environment
- Slips, Trips, and Falls
- Medical Gas Cylinder Storage
- Smoke-Free Policy
- Product Notices and Recalls

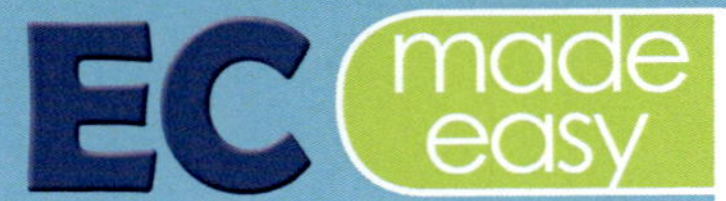

in other **words**

safety

The degree to which an intervention in the health care environment is free of risk for a patient and other persons, including workers. Safety risks may arise from the performance of tasks, from the structure of the physical environment, or from situations beyond the organization's control (such as weather).

safety and health management system (SHMS)

A systematic approach to managing safety and health activities by integrating occupational safety and health programs, policies, and objectives into organizational policies and procedures.

culture of safety

An environment in which safety is the top priority. In a culture of safety, not only are processes designed for optimal safety, but employees feel safe in reporting unsafe situations. Also referred to as a *safety culture.*

General Safety

Accidents, injuries, and illnesses: They're inevitable without effective safety precautions. These precautions include safety management plans and risk assessments that incorporate environmental tours (*see* Chapter 2). These should ideally be part of an overall program or system for general safety in your organization.

Safety and Health Management System (SHMS)

The Occupational Safety and Health Administration (OSHA) has a set of useful suggestions for a safety and health management system (SHMS). These align, in general, with Joint Commission standards related to the environment of care within an organization's overall safety program.

SHMS elements: Elements for an effective SHMS include the following:

- **Management leadership:** Ongoing and visible commitment and support from managers and executive-level leaders who establish a safety and health (S&H) policy, set goals, assign responsibilities, provide program evaluation, and evaluate safety records
- **Employee involvement:** Engagement of employees from every level in committees and groups as well as safety rules development, incident investigations, and peer training
- **Worksite analysis:** Comprehensive and regular evaluation of hazards and potential hazards (risks) in the workplace environment
- **Hazard prevention and control:** Procedures for identifying, correcting, and controlling hazards (perhaps involving a hierarchy of controls, such as engineering, work practice, and administrative controls)
- **Safety and health training:** Provision of safety and health training to employees
- **Accident/incident investigation:** Use of incident and accident investigation reports that answer who, what, where, when, and how
- **Safety culture:** Sustained implementation of a culture of safety, or safety culture, supported by top management

COLLABORATION: To make an SHMS work, everyone must work together. Accreditation professionals, you should be alert to all SHMS system activities related to compliance efforts. Safety officers and facilities directors, you should make sure all system approaches work efficiently and effectively across the entire organization—in all departments and all facilities. Leaders, you should be as involved as possible to demonstrate support and increase awareness. In particular, you should work with all levels of staff and managers to maintain a culture of safety, as defined in the Leadership (LD) standards.

High Reliability

Even though accidents, injuries, and illnesses do happen, your health care organization should strive to be a high reliability organization (HRO)—one that has succeeded in avoiding such adverse events in an environment where they might be expected to occur. For an organization to become an HRO, leadership must commit to that goal. Leaders must also work to implement and nurture an organizational culture that supports high reliability.

in other words

high reliability organization (HRO)
An organization that has fewer than its share of adverse events even while operating under stressful conditions.

KEY CONCEPT
Worker Safety

The way workers work may not be the right way. That includes the way workers interact with the environment—including the way they handle patients. Worker and patient safety go hand in hand. Fatigued clinical engineers may make errors in equipment repair that result in harm to patients. Caregivers who fail to use proper lifting equipment and techniques can easily injure themselves and patients they're trying to lift.

Worker safety requirements: It's not specified in Joint Commission standards, but worker safety should be woven throughout your risk management plans and performance improvement initiatives. And you should make it part of staff training. In addition, carefully follow OSHA standards to help reduce injuries and illnesses.

smart questions:

How is worker safety a part of your staff orientation and ongoing training?

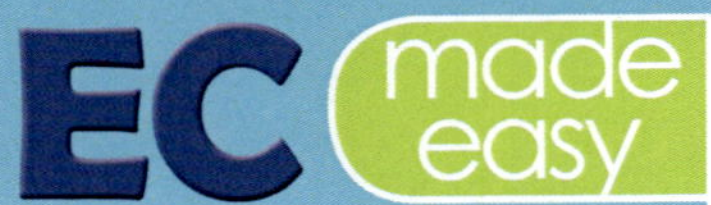

A Healthy Environment

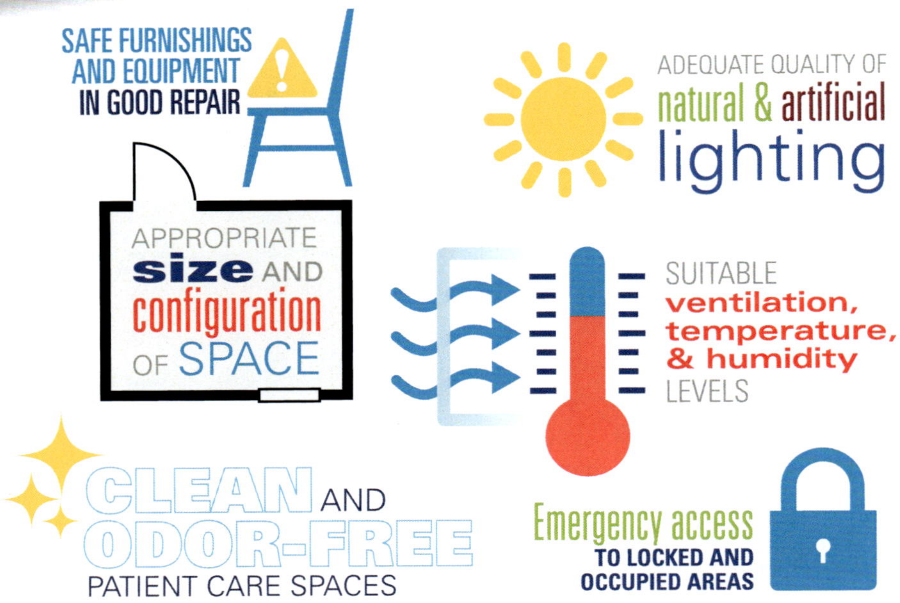

The physical environment of your health care organization should promote good health. And, of course, it must be able to meet the needs of the patient population(s) and the care, treatment, and services your organization provides. These features are addressed by one broad EC standard regarding providing a safe, functional environment.

A cost-effective concern: Keeping workers healthy in a health care environment just makes sense. But it can better safeguard an organization's bottom line as well. Keeping everyone safe decreases lost work time, injury compensation claims, and lawsuits. And it increases worker and patient satisfaction and staff retention.

in other words

ergonomics

Relating to how the worker "fits" with his or her tasks, work environment, and the equipment needed to get the job done properly.

Ergonomics

Worker safety requires an understanding of ergonomics. In terms of worker safety, this is about how the worker "fits" with his or her tasks, work environment, and the equipment needed to get the job done *correctly and safely* as well as efficiently.

Increased ergonomic risk: Tasks requiring the following can increase ergonomic risk:

- Repetitive, forceful, or prolonged exertions of the hands
- Frequent or heavy lifting and pushing, pulling, or carrying heavy objects
- Prolonged awkward postures
- Extended exposure to cold and vibration

Reduced ergonomic risk: Effective ergonomic practices and use of ergonomic equipment reduce these risks, especially the likelihood of musculoskeletal pain, stiffness, strains, and other injuries—many of which are caused by lifting and moving patients improperly. Involving staff in the selection of equipment and providing sufficient training are essential as well, of course.

Workarounds

There's no getting around it: Workarounds are going to happen. They happen when workflow and work processes aren't in synch. And when they happen, risk of injury (and worse) to workers and others can arise and persist to the point of crisis. That means you need to assess and monitor for potential workarounds.

Workaround factors: Consider these factors that contribute to workarounds:

- **Technology/equipment:** In health care, there's plenty of complicated technology and equipment. And there's always something "new." Ironically, failure to understand workflows as well as the impact of introducing something "new" into them can promote workarounds. Those workarounds often bypass safety features designed into "improved" systems.
- **Workload, fatigue, and distraction:** An inappropriate mix of staffing levels and an imbalance in workload assignments may lead overworked staff to take shortcuts. And the negative consequences of worker fatigue and distraction are well documented.

COLLABORATION: Having a well-rested, well-balanced, well-trained, and focused workforce should be a priority. Accreditation professionals and facilities directors, you can work with human resources personnel to make sure you have

Do your workers have access to appropriate ergonomic equipment that can prevent injuries? Have they been trained on its use?

in other words

workarounds

Alternative, informally designed, and inconsistently applied work processes that expedite workflow but sometimes subvert specific safeguards designed to prevent risk.

appropriate staffing and to develop worker safety training. And don't forget to involve frontline staff in any improvement efforts; they can provide valuable insight into issues affecting them. Leaders, you can support such efforts by providing sufficient resources.

Infection in the Environment

No health care organization can ignore infection prevention and control (IPC). Increasingly powerful and drug-resistant pathogens, including toxic strains of *Clostridium difficile*, as well as pandemic-potential diseases like influenza viruses, continue to pose dangers and require intensive efforts to prevent their growth and spread.

EC and IPC Safety Risks

The Joint Commission requires organizations to have an IPC program that includes risk assessment. Many of those risks have an intersection with the physical environment. This connection is evident in cross-references between the EC standards and Infection Prevention and Control (IC) standards. Following are some of the common safety areas where EC and IPC intersect:

- **Utilities:** The potential for airborne and waterborne infections via ventilation and water systems (*see* Chapter 6)
- **Emergency response:** Lack of clean water and other safeguards in the community during emergencies, which can lead to an influx of infectious patients, or pandemics (*see* Chapter 8)
- **Stick injuries:** Worker injuries from contaminated needles and other sharp instruments, collectively known as "sharps," which may occur during procedures as well as during room cleaning or linen removal (*see* the sidebar "Avoiding Injury and Infection from Sharps" on page 41)
- **Rooms and equipment:** Lack of proper cleaning and disinfecting of room surfaces (including the changing of curtains if they're visibly soiled) as well as equipment (particularly shared and reusable equipment, such as intravenous [IV] pumps) prior to or after them from an infected patient's room

in other words

sharps

Medical instruments (such as scalpels or hypodermic needles) that are sharp or may produce sharp pieces by shattering.

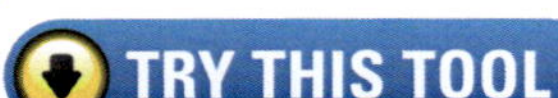

Environmental Services Checklists: Cleaning of Patient Rooms

Use these checklists to monitor proper daily cleaning and disinfecting of patient rooms.

- **PPE:** Failure of workers to wear the necessary personal protective equipment (PPE), or wear it correctly, to protect themselves against hazards in the environment, including bloodborne pathogens (BBPs)
- **Signage:** Lack of proper signage outside doors of rooms that carry a higher risk of transmission of microorganisms/infections
- **Staff training:** Lack of sufficient staff training in IPC practices
- **Staff immunization:** Poor staff immunization

Avoiding Injury and Infection from Sharps

Injuries caused by needles and other sharp instruments occur every day in health care organizations. If these "sharps" are contaminated, dangerous pathogens can be transmitted. The following strategies may help to reduce the risk of sharps injuries:

- Assess your health care organization's risks and injury experience through a review of available reports, injury surveillance, and staff surveys.
- Employ safe needle disposal methods and materials, including sharps disposal containers (*see* Chapter 5).
- Use blunt suture needles instead of sharp ones and use safety-engineered instruments.
- Implement a systematic approach to bloodborne pathogen (BBP) exposure prevention (as required by the Occupational Safety and Health Administration [OSHA]), including employee education programs, policies, and procedures to support injury prevention, reporting, and postexposure protocols.

KEY CONCEPT

Slips, Trips, and Falls

A slip, trip, and fall (STF) injury can happen anywhere to anyone. It can happen any time there's an unexpected change in contact between a person's feet and the flooring surface. Although most walking surfaces in health care facilities are slip-resistant when dry and clean, floor contaminants such as water, body fluids, or grease can easily lead to someone taking a spill. In patient homes, rugs and carpets are often trip culprits. And patients or persons with disabilities may be at greater risks of STF injuries due to their health conditions.

---

smart questions:

What types of PPE do your staff wear for daily cleaning? Who checks the condition of this PPE and how often?

in other words

personal protective equipment (PPE)

Equipment worn to minimize exposure to serious workplace injuries and illnesses that may result from contact with chemical, radiological, physical, electrical, mechanical, or other workplace hazards. PPE may include gloves, safety glasses, shoes, earplugs or muffs, hard hats, respirators, coveralls, vests, and full body suits.

smart questions:

Where are sharps disposal containers located and how and when are they emptied?

Medical Gas Considerations in Home Care

The organization delivering the gases is responsible for storing the cylinders of medical gases (or dewars of liquid oxygen) safely in the patient's home. This does not mean merely "dropping off" the cylinders. The organization must ensure that, at a minimum, medical gas cylinders are stored away from a source of heat, in a well-ventilated area, and in a manner that prevents them from falling over. Patient homes obviously are not subject to The Joint Commission's enforcement of the NFPA *Life Safety Code®*, but many elements of current good practice and common sense do apply.

Durable medical equipment (DME) companies, providers of respiratory equipment, and clinicians providing clinical respiratory care must identify risks associated with home oxygen therapy, such as fires. Consider the following three main elements:

(continued on page 44)

smart questions:

How are the empty and full freestanding medical gas cylinders labeled and segregated in your organization?

STF Risk Locations

Every area in a health care organization is susceptible to STF injuries, but the following are especially troublesome:

- **Food service areas:** Kitchens, cafeterias, lounges, patient rooms, and any other areas where food is prepared, served, consumed, and cleaned up
- **Bathrooms:** Tubs, showers, and around toilets and sinks in inpatient or resident rooms and in patients' home bathrooms
- **Specialized areas:** Emergency and operating rooms, pharmacy, and radiology
- **Outdoor areas:** Parking garages, walkways, and entrances/exits

STF risk assessment and monitoring: As you might expect, STF risks should be included in your safety risk assessments. Careful monitoring should be spelled out in your management plans. Condition of floor surface, type of floor surface (tile, slip-resistant flooring, carpet), as well as the presence of adequate lighting, handrails, and grab bars should be checked as part of environmental rounds and tours (*see* Chapter 2).

KEY CONCEPT

Medical Gas Cylinder Storage

Sometimes it's impractical to have piped nonflammable medical gases in a health care setting. In those cases, the organization provides the gases in freestanding cylinders. Make sure to follow hospital policy when handling and using freestanding cylinders. If an empty cylinder is delivered to a patient, it could have serious patient care consequences. Thus, these requirements:

- Stored freestanding medical gas cylinders (including oxygen tanks), must be labeled and safe to use on a patient.
- Empty cylinders must be physically segregated from all other cylinders and clearly labeled as "empty."

Labeling Cylinders

You should clearly label which cylinders are full and which are empty. The Joint Commission leaves it to the individual organization to determine how to do this marking.

- **Full vs. empty?:** What constitutes a "full" cylinder vs. an "empty" one? The Joint Commission allows organizations to determine what constitutes an empty or full cylinder. The organization should work with nursing and respiratory care to define how they will manage compressed gas cylinders. This must be defined in policy or procedure so it is clear to staff when using, handling, or storing compressed gas cylinders. The use of clearly worded, color-coded labels, such as those below will facilitate proper handling and management.

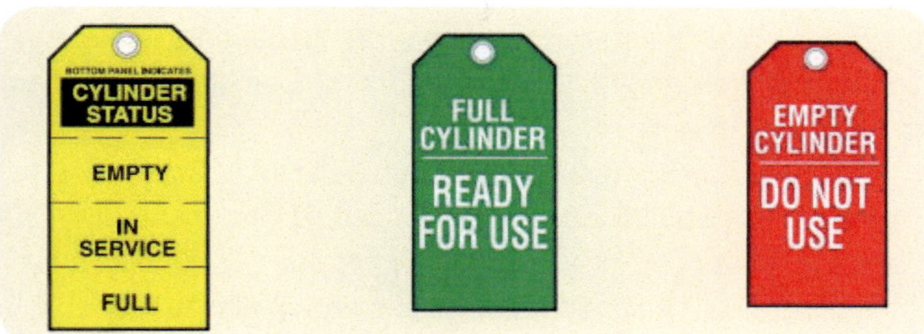

Separating Cylinders

You must physically segregate (separate) empty and full cylinders in one of these ways:

- **Separate racks:** Storing empty and full cylinders in separate, marked racks
- **Physical barriers:** Using physical barriers to separate empty and full cylinders
- **Color-coding:** Distinguishing empty and full cylinders by color-coding the storage racks
- **Other:** Employing other effective means of physically separating empty and full cylinders

An organization could have a "full" rack and an "empty" rack. Or, in one rack, it might have a "patient ready" row, and an "in service" or "in use" row, and an "empty" row, as long as each category of cylinder is segregated from each other. For example, you'd be fine if you had a rack where the first row is colored green and labeled "full," the next two rows are colored yellow and labeled "partial," and the fourth row is colored red and labeled "empty."

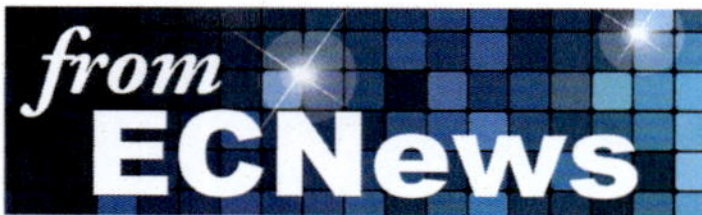

(continued from page 42)

1. A home safety risk assessment that includes evaluating, at least, the presence of smoking materials and other fire safety risks and checking to ensure that there are functioning smoke detectors

2. A process for informing the patient, family members, and caregivers of the findings of the safety risk assessment

3. A process for educating those individuals about the specific recommendations made based on the risk assessment

The organizations are also required to assess these individuals' comprehension of, as well as their ability and willingness to comply with, the recommended interventions.

—adapted from "Medical Gases: Tips for Safe Use and Storage," by George Mills, Director of the Department of Engineering at The Joint Commission, *Environment of Care® News*, December 2012

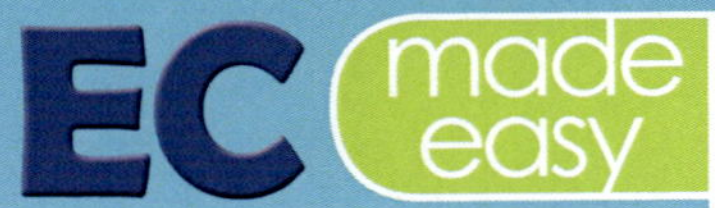

Smoke-Free Policy

Supporting good health is what your organization is all about. And everyone knows that smoking is bad for your health. Not only that, but one of the biggest risks to a facility is a lit cigarette or other combustible smoking product. That's why organizations today are adopting smoke-free policies (SFPs) and tobacco cessation programs (TCPs).

More Reasons to Be Smoke-Free

Putting a smoke-free policy in place protects patients, staff, and visitors from the dangers of secondhand smoke. It also satisfies two EC requirements:

- That organizations develop a written policy prohibiting smoking in all buildings (except in specific circumstances) and maintain compliance with this policy
- That organizations manage fire risks and minimize the potential for harm caused by fire, smoke, and other products of combustion (*see* Chapter 7)

E-cigarettes: Make sure your policy addresses electronic cigarettes (e-cigarettes). They don't contain tobacco or require a match or lighter to ignite—but they still pose a fire hazard because they involve a source of ignition (*see* the sidebar "E-Cigarettes as an Ignition Source" below).

E-Cigarettes as an Ignition Source

E-cigarettes utilize a battery to send a small electrical current to a device, called an atomizer, which vaporizes a nicotine solution to be inhaled by the user. To vaporize the liquid, the atomizer must convert the electrical current into heat, which can present a fire hazard. Although this is a significantly lower fire risk than in tobacco-burning cigarettes, it is still a risk.

In addition, many of these portable devices include a rechargeable battery; malfunctions, including explosions and fires, have occurred with these batteries and their charger units. (To avoid the risk of fire, an e-cigarette user should be cognizant of when the e-cigarette battery may become activated unintentionally; left unchecked, such activation can overheat the atomizer and pose a fire risk. Also, cheap and incompatible charger units should never be used.

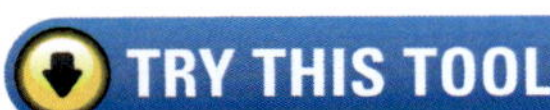

Smoke-Free Policy Development Checklist
This checklist suggests action steps to take in creating a smoke-free policy or evaluating an existing one.

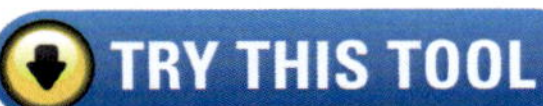

Smoke-Free Policy Scripts
Use these scripts to train employees on how to approach smokers about your smoke-free policy.

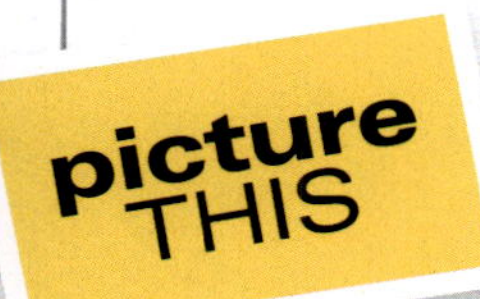

Smoke-Free Signage

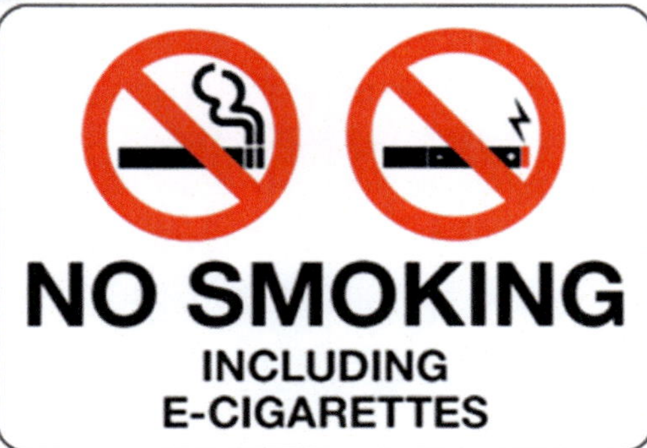

Posting signs at and within the borders of your smoke-free zone will help smokers to self-regulate. Use a strong visual symbol in addition to any written statements to make sure everyone understands your message clearly.

KEY CONCEPT

Product Notices and Recalls

Few things compromise the safety of patients and staff as much as a defective product that can fail or malfunction when you least expect it. So pay attention to product notices and recalls issued by manufacturers. You might find out about these alerts from physicians, from administrators, from the manufacturers themselves, and/or from suppliers or vendors.

Responding to Alerts

Regardless of how you find out about the alert, your organization must have a clear process for responding to it—a process all staff members should be familiar with. Here are some tips:

- **Put a response process in the plan:** Define a process for responding to notices and recalls—and put it in your safety management plan (*see* Chapter 2). In this process, include information about the following:
  - Who should review the alerts and how to check them against products actually in use in your organization

smart questions:

What is your process for responding to product notices and recalls?

- How to notify appropriate departments about the alert
- What department staff should do in response to the notification
- An expected turnaround time for resolution of the alert
- How to document the response process
- **Put a communication process into effect:** Establish a communication process with manufacturers, suppliers, and vendors so that the right person(s) in your organization is automatically alerted whenever there's a notice or recall. (Note: Medication recalls are covered under Joint Commission Medication Management [MM] standards.)

TOOLS OF THE TRADE

- Work Flow Assessment Checklist
- Environmental Services Checklists: Cleaning of Patient Rooms
- Smoke-Free Policy Development Checklist
- Smoke-Free Policy Scripts

CHAPTER 4
Security

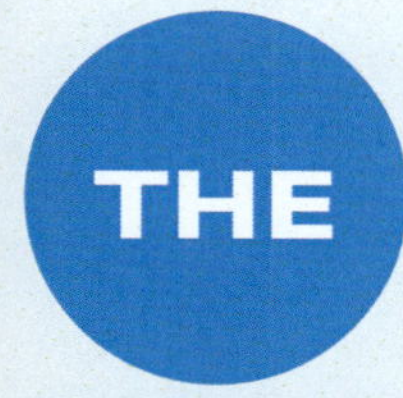
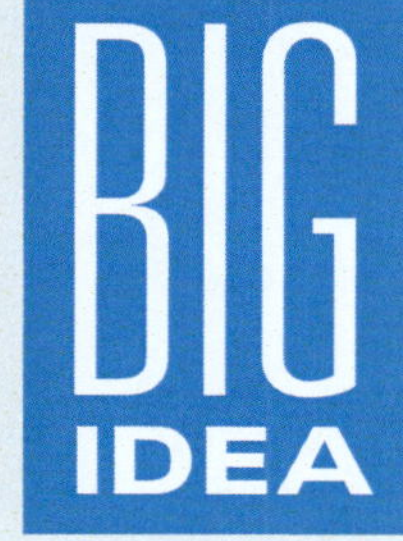

Health care shootings. The threat of terrorism. Infant abduction and civil unrest. Every health care organization in business today has to protect against headline-grabbing security issues such as these. But security is about protecting your organization from more common threats too, including drug theft, patient suicide, and wandering patients. Security risks of all kinds are related to incidents that are often *intentional* and result in harm or loss to people and property. That's why security is also about making staff, patients, family, and visitors feel secure—and making sure the fact matches the feeling.

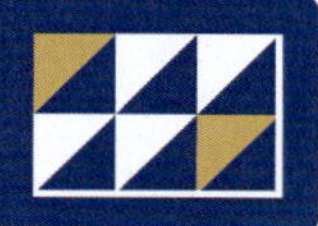

THE MANUAL

Following are the relevant Joint Commission *Comprehensive Accreditation Manual* (*CAM*) chapters:

- Environment of Care (EC)
- Leadership (LD)

KEY CONCEPTS

- Access Control
- Abductions and Elopements
- Environmental Suicide Risks
- Workplace Violence
- Security Incident Reporting
- Security Risk Assessment and Analysis

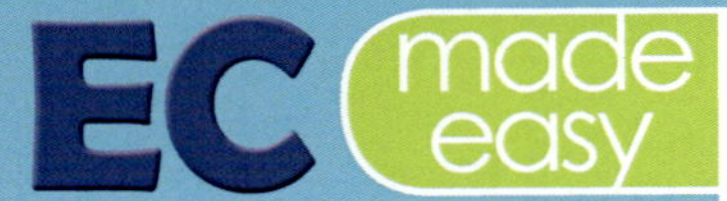

in other words

access control

The management of admission to areas within a facility based on permission levels assigned to users. Access control often includes authentication of the identity of the user.

KEY CONCEPT

Access Control

Your organization's first step in making sure patients, staff, and equipment in a facility are protected—and feel protected—is setting up access control protocols. Essentially, this is about determining who needs access to where and denying access to those who don't have clearance.

Determining Access Needs

The big challenges in controlling access involve doing it without interfering in patient care and complying with the *Life Safety Code®*.* To strike that balance, you should review staff responsibilities to determine who needs access to what areas. Also consider patients, visitors, and contract employees, and what areas they can and can't enter. This helps to contain access (limiting it to those who need it).

COLLABORATION: Leaders who are unit directors or department managers, you understand best how your areas run. So facilities or securities directors, why not call on them to assist with making decisions about containing access? Close the loop and provide feedback when the *Life Safety Code* prohibits implementing changes a department manager or director would like. Accreditation professionals, you can solicit feedback by conducting tracers that assess how well access controls are working in an area.

Controlling Access with Identification

The standards for most organizations require identifying people entering a facility. You can do this by simple visual surveillance, or for more controlled areas, by using authentication devices. Authentication devices prove the identity of a person requesting access. Those who need identification are listed here, with typical authentication devices:

- **Inpatients:** Inpatients often wear identification wristbands, but in nursing care centers and some behavioral facilities, that may not be common practice.
- **Visitors and contract employees:** Organizations usually keep track of visitors and contract employees in facilities by having them sign in and out at the reception desk.

Temporary identification cards or badges are also common. Many organizations are also using photo visitor passes—a process that includes scanning the visitor's driver's license.

- **Staff:** Staff attire, such as lab coats or scrubs, is not a safe method of staff identification; impostors can easily get hold of clothing like that. Many organizations use a photo ID card system with a card reader or smart cards with assigned access rights. (Note: Some states regulate the use of ID badges and what needs to be on them.)

Access to Security-Sensitive Areas

Here's a sensitive subject—at least in terms of security: security-sensitive areas. Joint Commission Environment of Care (EC) standards require you to manage security risks and control access to and from areas you designate as security sensitive. These areas are considered particularly vulnerable to security threats and require special access control protocols. Security-sensitive areas typically include those described below.

Pharmacy: Prescription drugs, especially controlled substances, are a lure for addicts and criminals. Armed robbery and drug diversion are the primary risks.

- **Addressing the risks:** A closed and locked pharmacy is the best protection. Limited service openings, protective glass, clear lines of sight to doors and corridors, panic buttons, and closed-circuit television cameras can all be life-saving security safeguards.

Emergency department: Crowding, long wait times, and anxiety about an urgent medical condition can make the emergency department (ED) a tense place, increasing the potential for violence. Patients with acute physical or psychological stress cause most ED security incidents. But you can't ask them to leave until they've been evaluated and treated, if necessary.

- **Addressing the risks:** Clear communication about waiting times can ease frustration. But ED staff need training in dealing with aggressors. Simulations of potential security threats can help prep for the stress of the real thing.

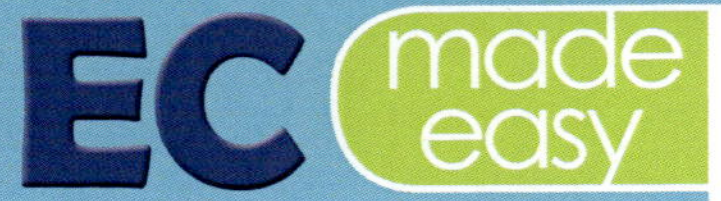

Additional areas: Other areas that organizations may choose to designate as security sensitive include these:

- Maternity and infant care units
- Intensive care units
- Radiology departments
- Parking facilities
- Medical records department
- Cashier offices
- Behavioral health care units
- Specialized outpatient clinics (substance abuse, abortion)
- Operating room, neonatal intensive care unit, postanesthesia care unit

Access Control Plan

To make sure everyone is on the same page about access control, you might want to have a written access control plan in addition to your security management plan (*see* Chapter 2).

Control plan activities: This plan would cover the following main activities:

- **Denying access:** Establishing who isn't allowed where and when
- **Containing access:** Identifying who is allowed where and why (which might incorporate a clearance-level system)
- **Controlling access:** Describing how access is controlled, including identification methods as well as security equipment and protocols, such as monitoring and securing entry and exit points to security-sensitive areas
- **Documenting movement:** Spelling out your recordkeeping requirements (sign-in/out records, surveillance records, and so on)

KEY CONCEPT

Abductions and Elopements

In the simplest terms:
- Abductions occur when patients are taken from a health care facility without permission.
- Elopements occur when patients wander off or leave an around-the-clock facility unsupervised or without permission.

In many organizations, these events generally involve patients who are vulnerable to harm (infants, children, and the elderly).

For that reason, they require a swift security team response that may involve community law enforcement. In behavioral health care organizations, however, elopements generally involve adults who don't want to continue treatment and aren't particularly vulnerable to harm.

Infant and Child Abduction

Most abductions from health care facilities involve infants and children. And it isn't always patients who are abducted; it can be visitors too. The risk for abductions must be taken seriously, even though abductions don't happen often (and when they do, victims are usually recovered).

Abduction response: Staff members are usually the first to discover that an infant or child is missing. Security is then notified immediately. This is followed quickly by an announcement via the public address system of a specific code for an infant or child abduction (for example, "Code Pink + 1 + male/female"), which initiates a critical incident response. After the code is delivered, the organization mobilizes in the response effort, with staff performing preassigned tasks as rapidly as possible.

Written response plan: The National Center for Missing & Exploited Children (NCMEC) offers helpful strategies and recommends that every health care facility develop a written response plan for infant abductions. And Joint Commission standards require hospitals and critical access hospitals to have written procedures to follow in the handling of an infant or pediatric abduction. You can make that part of your security management plan or you can have a separate document referenced in the plan (*see* Chapter 2). Of course, you need to share any response plans with all staff members in infant and child care areas and provide response training.

Abduction security tools: Tools an organization can use to address infant and child abduction risks include the following:

- **Infant and mother identification systems:** This might include systems such as band matching, DNA identification, and antibody profiles.
- **Restricted access devices:** These include card readers, access-controlled egress, and delayed egress devices.

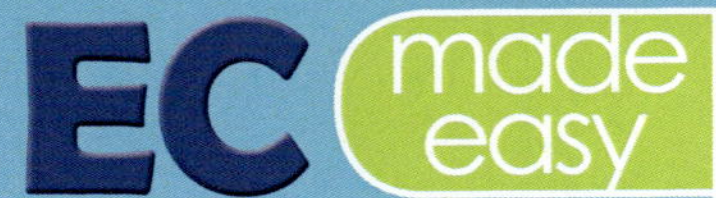

- **Video cameras and surveillance:** Although cameras may serve as a deterrent, they must be functioning to be effective in an actual event. Video surveillance—including remote monitoring—saves money as well as lives by reducing the need for on-site security staff in every area of the facility.
- **Tagging mechanisms:** This might be a band attached to the infant's or child's ankle, wrist, or umbilical cord. Movement past any of the strategically located sensors triggers an alarm.
- **Staff and parent education:** Making everyone—including parents—aware of security systems is paramount to avoid both real threats and false alarms.

Pediatric and Geriatric Elopements

Both children and the elderly are prone to elopement. These patients typically require a level of supervision to remain safe, so elopement can be dangerous. Dangers can include being injured by traffic, drowning in open water, falling from a high place, unintended encounters with people with harmful intentions, and exposure to foul weather or environmental conditions, resulting in hypothermia, heat stroke, or dehydration.

Child elopement: Children with special needs are especially at risk of eloping. They may be trying to leave because they're scared or overwhelmed. Often they hide in or are drawn to places that interest them—including places outside the facility that may be dangerous. Children without special needs are also at risk of eloping, of course; many children are naturally curious. And some children may just be trying to go home.

Geriatric elopement: Patient elopement is a risk in the geriatric or Alzheimer's units of a health care organization. Wandering off is not uncommon for geriatric patients who are physically capable but mentally impaired (as a result of Alzheimer's disease or another form of dementia or who may be disoriented as a result of a drug).

COLLABORATION: Your organization should respond quickly to any elopement to prevent harm to the patient. But who's going to respond in what ways? You need to work together to have a cohesive, comprehensive, and cooperative response plan.

Leaders at the executive level, you'll likely talk to media. Clinical leaders and security personnel, you'll talk to the family and coordinate the search assignments among staff as well as local police, if they need to be called in. Accreditation professionals, you'll probably work with facilities directors: You two will make sure the response follows the approved procedures outlined in your security management plan, as required by Joint Commission standards.

KEY CONCEPT

Environmental Suicide Risks

All health care environments should be as safe, humane, and therapeutic as possible. A safe health care environment is one that's free of dangerous materials or structures that could aid a patient in a suicide attempt. Many suicidal patients suffer from depression, schizophrenia, or other mental disorders, so organizations treating such patients are obviously at the greatest risk. But it can also be a risk in nonbehavioral health care units and EDs, areas with increasing suicide incidents, as documented in *Sentinel Event Alert*, Issue 46.

Suicide Risks and Responses

Your risk assessments (*see* Chapter 2), including any EC rounds or tours, should identify potential suicide risks in the environment. The number of possible items and ligature points used in suicide attempts aren't limitless but are plentiful enough to require a checklist or other tool to ensure thoroughness on routine reviews.

An environmental response: Suicide prevention may require changes to patient rooms and limits on patient access to supplies or equipment. Approaches for reducing threats can range from simple or inexpensive solutions to more robust environmental design changes. Your organization may want to consider doing the following:

- Replace glass windows and glass in artwork framing with polycarbonate or acrylic material.
- Replace or fortify removable ceiling tiles.
- Cover exposed plumbing.
- Employ technologies and products to make the space more secure, including tamper-proof screws, antiligature handrails and fixtures, breakaway bars, fixed furniture, cordless beds, and so on.

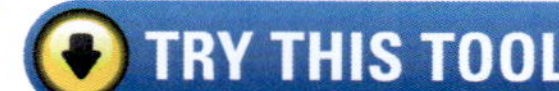

Environmental Risks for Suicide Assessment Checklist
This checklist will help you address suicide risks in the nonbehavioral health units and emergency departments.

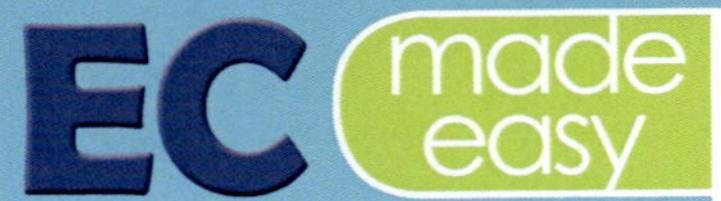

Possible Items and Ligature Points Used in Suicide Attempts

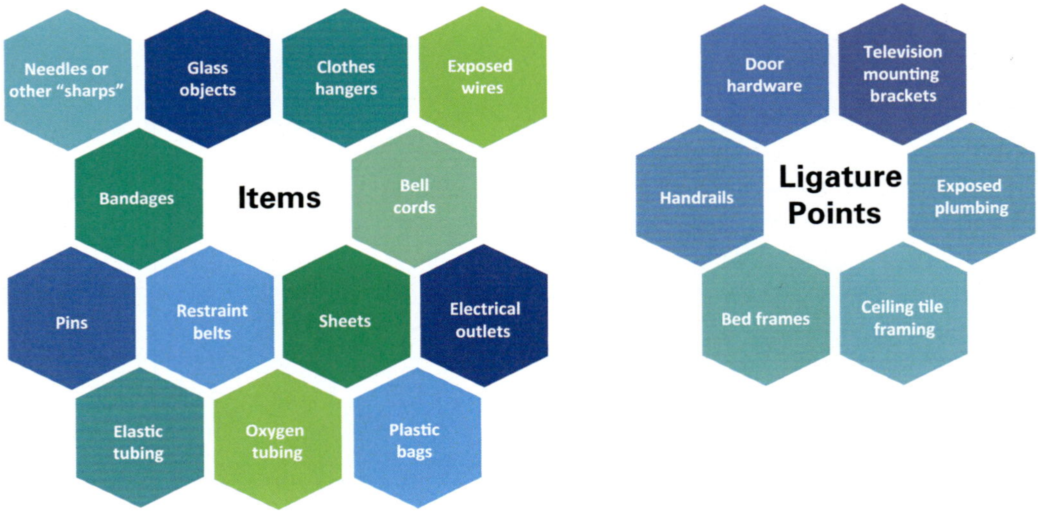

COLLABORATION: If you're a facilities director, evaluate all environmental response options for potential benefit—based on your organization's risk assessment. If any of the risks compromise compliance to Joint Commission standards, talk to your accreditation professional right away before any situations escalate to an immediate threat (*see* Chapter 2). Together with leaders and others involved in performance improvement (PI), you can formulate a plan that prioritizes repairs or alterations. If high-risk hazards in an area can't be fixed right away, you'll need to work with clinical unit leaders to make sure at-risk patients located there are supervised directly. *See* the sidebar "Sample Risk Assessment: Exposed Plumbing in a Behavioral Unit" below for an example of how a risk assessment might look. It follows the standardized risk assessment format outlined in Chapter 2.

An educational response: Your organization can also reduce suicide risks through staff education and training. Make sure staff members understand environmental risks for suicide, how to identify those risks, how to report them, and how to prevent them. For example, all staff should be alert at all times for potentially dangerous objects.

smart questions:

Are clinical and environmental services staff in your organization trained in awareness of environmental risks for suicide? Are leaders?

Sample Risk Assessment: Exposed Plumbing in a Behavioral Unit

➤ **Step 1 — Identify the issue:** Whether or not to allow exposed plumbing in a behavioral health unit.

➤ **Step 2 — List advantages:**
- We have no history of adverse events associated with exposed plumbing.
- We have clinical interventions in place to prevent patient self-harm even with pipes present.
- We could instead designate "high-risk" rooms that don't have exposed plumbing, and have patients move from a high-risk to a low-risk room as treatment progresses.

➤ **Step 3 — List disadvantages:**
- Exposed plumbing presents opportunities for patient self-harm.
- If a clinical intervention fails, how do we prevent patient self-harm?

➤ **Step 4 — Evaluate both sides:** Discuss among all stakeholders, including unit physicians and nursing staff, risk management, facilities, and administration.

➤ **Step 5 — Reach a conclusion:** Decide whether to allow exposed plumbing in a behavioral health unit.

➤ **Step 6 — Document the process:** Share the decision with the EC committee, using the report as documentation. Update relevant policies or procedures, if needed.

➤ **Step 7 — Monitor and reassess:** Review incident reports related to patient self-harm for three months. Then revisit the issue:
- If the decision is valid based on the data, revisit it annually.
- If the decision is not valid, conduct the risk assessment process again.

KEY CONCEPT

Workplace Violence

- According to the US Occupational Safety and Health Administration (OSHA), nearly two million American workers report having been victims of workplace violence each year, with many more cases going unreported.
- According to The Joint Commission's Sentinel Event Database, assault, rape, or homicide are among the most commonly reviewed sentinel event types.

in other words

workplace violence

Any physical assault, threatening behavior, or verbal abuse occurring in the workplace setting.

Motivated by these facts, both OSHA and The Joint Commission advocate that health care organizations have a written and comprehensive workplace violence prevention program. OSHA inspects organizations after complaints or incidents of workplace violence. And, although Joint Commission standards don't include specific requirements for workplace violence prevention, they do require you to manage safety and security risks. Workplace violence is a significant risk.

Workplace Violence: Who, What, Where, and When

Workplace violence can affect many individuals, cover a variety of acts, and occur in a broad range of areas under untold conditions. As noted above, it's widespread, and by most accounts, it's increasing in scope and severity.

Perpetrators and victims: Workplace violence perpetrators and victims may be anyone: staff, patients, or visitors—both internal and external:

- **Internal:** Staff, patients, or visitors may threaten other staff, patients, or visitors. In any case, remember that safety for staff—including contract workers—is just as important as safety for patients and visitors. Any threats to anyone should be reported to security immediately.
- **External:** Some staff, patients, or visitors may be in danger from someone outside your organization, such as current or past spouses/partners or someone connected with a crime or conflict, including gang members. If your organization learns of such a threat, everyone involved with the person under threat should be made aware of the potential for violence to increase vigilance.

Varieties of violence: Workplace violence can take many forms, but it generally falls into two broad categories:

- **Verbal violence:** This may occur in person or by phone/text or postings on the Internet. It includes threats (to inflict bodily harm, including vague or hidden threats), harassment (such as shouting and abusive or offensive language, gestures, or other discourteous conduct), and accusations (making false, malicious, or unfounded statements against someone with the intention of damaging that person's reputation or undermining authority). Attempts to cause psychological trauma with verbal intimidation or other statements are also considered verbal violence.

- **Physical violence:** This encompasses attempts to cause physical harm and actual acts of physical harm (stalking, striking, pushing, slapping, rape, beatings, shootings, stabbings). It also includes disorderly conduct (throwing or pushing objects, punching walls, slamming doors). It even includes suicide and attempted suicide, as that's physical violence against oneself. Terrorism, when the intention is to kill or make ill, falls under this category as well.

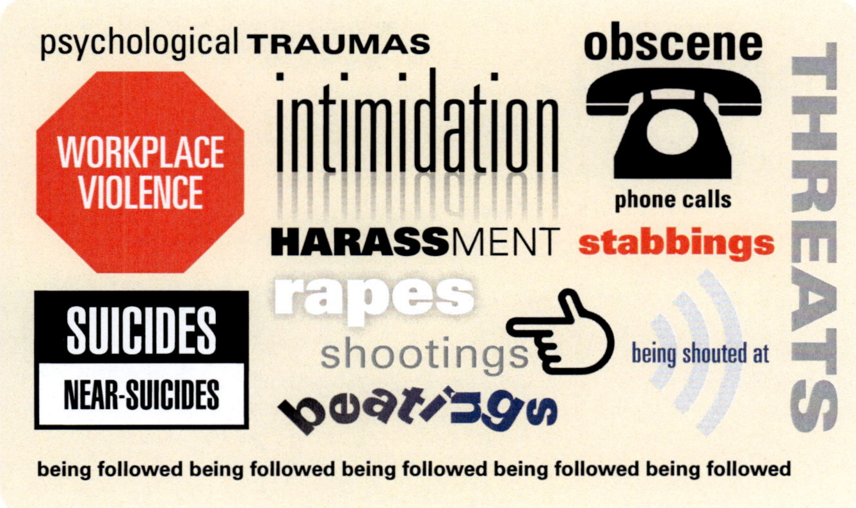

Any place, any time: Although violence may occur anywhere in a health care organization, it's most prevalent in psychiatric hospitals and psychiatric wards, EDs, waiting rooms, and geriatric care areas. In addition, employees who work alone during evening and night shifts (including home care staff who may work in dangerous neighborhoods) may be at high risk for workplace violence. In these situations, workers can be isolated and have a smaller pool of available staff nearby to assist in a potentially dangerous situation. Getting timely response to violent behavior is difficult—but vital—under these circumstances.

Stopping Workplace Violence

Violence in the workplace often happens randomly or without warning. Your organization can take the following actions to better prepare for, prevent, and respond to such incidents:

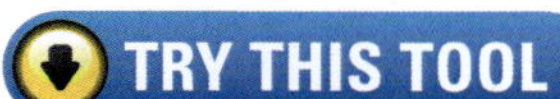
TRY THIS TOOL

Environmental Risks for Workplace Violence Checklist
This checklist features questions that will help your organization determine the environmental risk factors for workplace violence.

- **Put it in the plan:** In your security management plan (*see* Chapter 2), include workplace violence prevention strategies or a description of any program you have in place that addresses it.
- **Make it part of staff training:** Incorporate workplace violence as a topic in staff training, including training in de-escalation—managing disruptive and assaultive behaviors through verbal and nonverbal techniques (*see* the sidebar "Watch Out for Workplace Violence" below). Ideally, workplace violence training should be part of orientation of all employees.
- **Include it in policies and procedures:** Address workplace violence in appropriate policies and procedures, such as those on safety culture (*see* Chapter 3).
- **Consider physical changes in response to it:** Examine the potential need to restructure the physical environment (different parking lot lighting, barriers, and so on) to protect against workplace violence.

Watch Out for Workplace Violence

Staff training in workplace violence should be part of any workplace violence prevention program or risk reduction strategy. Following basic prevention principles and recognizing warning signs are an elementary part of this training.

Warning Signs

- Facially expressing anger or frustration
- Verbally expressing anger or frustration
- Using body language such as threatening gestures
- Presence of alcohol or other drugs
- Presence of a weapon, whether conventional (a knife or gun) or unconventional (something picked up from the health care environment)

Basic Principles

- Don't assume that being hurt is part of the job. It's not.
- Avoid being alone with a potentially violent person.
- Don't let the person get between you and the door or other escape route.
- Respond to the person calmly and with understanding.
- Use de-escalation techniques to help calm the person down.
- Don't overestimate your ability to handle the situation. If you know you can't handle it or see it escalating, leave and call security immediately.

COLLABORATION: Leaders, you need to make sure your organization is supporting a safety culture that ensures a secure, nonviolent environment for everyone in your organization (*see* Chapter 3). That means placing as much importance on employee safety and health as on serving patients. Accreditation professionals, you need to make sure leaders do that because it's required by The Joint Commission—and work together with leaders and security and safety officers on workplace violence education programs. Facilities directors, safety officers, or security directors, you need to make sure everyone understands and applies the security protocols in your security management plan. You also need to establish liaisons with law enforcement representatives and others who can show how to prevent or reduce aggressive behavior. Use OSHA's risk assessment to help identify risk.

An Active Shooter Situation

It's shocking, but shootings are one type of workplace violence becoming more frequent in health care settings. Knowing how to recognize and respond to an active shooter situation is now, unfortunately, a necessary part of health care staff training. This situation is one of various types of active threats that require immediate response.

The nature of an active shooter situation: Attacks like this are extremely hard to predict. An active shooter can be a patient, family member, staff member, or someone who isn't even associated with your organization. Most active shooter incidents end in minutes, often before the police arrive, so you need to be prepared to respond quickly.

Risk assessment for an active shooter situation: Make sure your organization includes an active shooter situation as part of your security plan risk assessment, especially if your health care setting is in an area with a high crime rate. Gauge your vulnerabilities regarding access and security measures such as cameras, door locks, and metal detectors.

Can your staff recognize warning signs of impending violence?

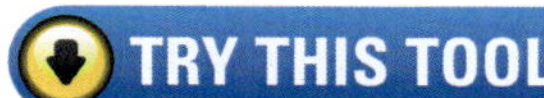

Pocket Card: Workplace Violence De-Escalation Strategies
This pocket card can help prepare staff for what to do in a workplace violence situation by providing de-escalation strategies.

in other words

active shooter
An individual actively engaged in killing or attempting to kill people in a confined and populated area; in most cases, active shooters use firearms, and there's no pattern or method to their selection of victims.

active threat
A situation that occurs without warning, quickly degenerates, and has the potential to cause death or serious injury.

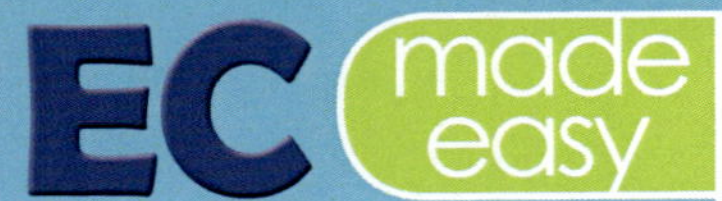

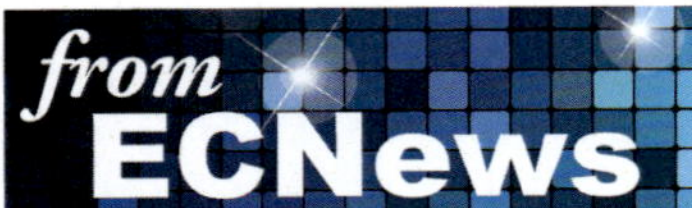

OSHA & Worker Safety: Assault Halt

Many effective tactics for responding to a violent incident can be taught to, practiced by, and executed by staff—particularly techniques such as effective blocking of punches and kicks; freeing yourself from grabs, choke holds, hair pulls, and bites; and maintaining a safe personal space buffer of three to six feet from a patient while providing care.

It's also crucial to have systems and procedures in place to summon help, barricade areas, and notify occupants of a violent event, such as panic buttons, lockdown mechanisms, and code orange alert notifications.

—excerpted from
"Assault Halt: OSHA and
The Joint Commission Offer
Guidance and Resources to Curb
Workplace Violence,"
Environment of Care® News,
April 2016

Preparing for an active shooter situation: Preparing for an active shooter situation means knowing what to do without having to "look it up." It means having a targeted response plan and drilling everyone on that plan. Most plans follow strategies that involve evacuation, hiding, calling for help, and, as a last resort, taking action against the shooter (*see* the sidebar "Active Shooter Response Plan" below).

Active Shooter Response Plan

Common strategies employed in most active shooter response plans are described below. Some organizations name the strategies in a way to create an easy-to-remember acronym, and/or create pocket cards to use in an active shooter situation.

Evacuate

If possible, immediately evacuate an area where a shooter is present—even if others don't want to follow. Leave all belongings. When police arrive and you're exiting the scene, keep your hands visible and elevated with open palms.

Hide

If evacuating isn't possible, hide, preferably in a room with doors that can be locked or blocked. Once in the room, make it look like it's empty by turning off lights and equipment and closing windows, curtains, or blinds. Then take cover under a large item, such as a desk, and stay still and quiet.

Call

After you're in a secure location, call for security or the police. This should be done only on a phone; shouting can alert the shooter to the location. If you aren't able to speak or text quietly, keep the line open for responders to listen in. Try to give the following information in as much detail as possible:
- Location of the incident
- Number of perpetrators
- Number of victims and any hostages
- Type and size of the weapon used by the shooter
- What's currently happening

Act

As a last resort, if you're in imminent danger and are unable to evacuate or hide, take action against the active shooter. This may be an attempt to disrupt or incapacitate the shooter by acting aggressively or by throwing items or improvised weapons.

KEY CONCEPT

Security Incident Reporting

Unusual events? Suspicious activity? Criminal behavior? In your workplace? Report it—and report it now. Reporting is a responsibility of all health care staff and should be done promptly. That's key to bringing about a swift resolution to an incident or potential incident.

A Reporting System

Chances are, your organization already has incident reporting forms. But does it have a reporting system? And does everyone know how to use those forms and that system?

Elements of a reporting system: It's not required, but it's a good idea to make sure your system has at least these elements spelled out:

- **What types of incidents are security incidents:** This might seem obvious, but is a staff person locked in a bathroom a security incident or not? It may help to list criteria for security incidents or explain types of security incidents. It might also help to classify them and give examples. Consider rating them by severity or criticality.
- **How to report a security incident:** What information is important to give for each type of incident? Which incidents can or should be reported by phone, radio, or in person? Are anonymous reports allowed? What forms need to be filled out? Is other documentation required, such as photos?
- **Who to contact to report an incident and when:** This might vary by type of incident or level of criticality. It needs to be clear. Do you report a particular incident to a security officer or your supervisor? Can a receptionist or operator decide whom to contact about an incident if you call the main number?
- **Who can report a security incident:** Basically, anyone should be able to report an incident, but completing certain incident forms may need to be done by managers or supervisors.
- **How incidents are analyzed:** Security incident report records should be examined by the EC committee (*see* Chapter 1) to identify trends or patterns for follow-up and possible changes. How often that should be done and how

to coordinate it as part of your monitoring activities should be part of your plan (*see* Chapter 2).

Reporting security incidents to The Joint Commission:
Depending on your organization, certain security incidents may be subject to review by The Joint Commission. These are typically sentinel events. You should check your accreditation manual, but such events include abduction, elopement, suicide, rape, assault, and murder under specific conditions.

Security Risk Analysis Form
You can use this security risk analysis form to help identify which security risks are most urgent.

KEY CONCEPT
Security Risk Assessment and Analysis

Risk assessment is a required part of your security management plan (*see* Chapter 2). It typically follows a cyclical process, with monitoring as a major component, especially for security risks. Risk analysis comes after the risk assessment: You have to rank and prioritize the risks you uncover: Which risks are most urgent to address first?

Involvement in Risk Assessment and Analysis
Risk assessment and analysis may be performed by the EC committee, with participation from an accreditation professional or risk manager. Others may—and probably should—be involved as well for various reasons:

- **Security staff:** To provide internal expertise
- **External security experts:** To establish a protection baseline and advise on challenging problems
- **Department managers:** To share related work flow and staffing issues
- **Staff members:** To offer their frontline perspective

COLLABORATION: Facilities director or security manager, you should be mindful of how security risks dovetail with other EC risks across the organization and/or health care system. Leaders, you should ask for periodic reports on any contracted security experts to assess their performance and value, per

Joint Commission standards. Accreditation professionals, you should review risk assessments too and meet with leaders and the facilities director, especially if there are situations that require immediate action for maintaining accreditation.

TOOLS OF THE TRADE

- Environmental Risks for Suicide Assessment Checklist
- Environmental Risks for Workplace Violence Checklist
- Pocket Card: Workplace Violence De-Escalation Strategies
- Security Risk Analysis Form

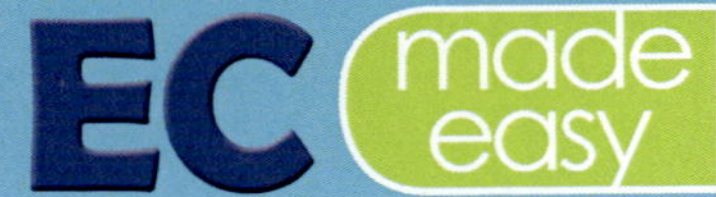

CHAPTER 5

Hazardous Materials and Waste

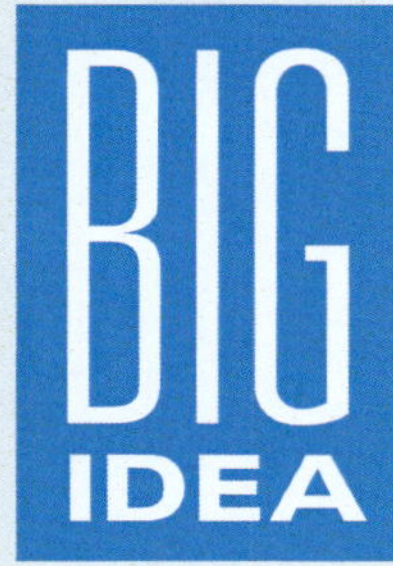

Bloodborne pathogens, radioactive waste, hazardous vapors, and hazardous energy sources, such as radiation, lasers, and microwaves. These are present in many health care environments. It may seem ironic to have hazardous materials in a health care organization. But with careful management, many of these materials, such as chemotherapeutic drugs and bleach, can benefit patients and help keep your physical environment clean and safe. The commitment for managing hazardous materials and waste (or hazmat) is "from cradle to grave." In other words, you have to manage hazardous materials and waste from the time they enter any facility in your organization to the time they're finally shipped out of your facility and disposed of. That means you need to think through and be prepared for the many risks surrounding these materials to ensure the safety of patients, staff, visitors, and the community.

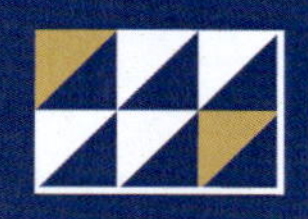

THE MANUAL

Following are the relevant Joint Commission *Comprehensive Accreditation Manual (CAM)* chapters:

- Environment of Care (EC)
- Leadership (LD)
- Infection Prevention and Control (IC)

KEY CONCEPTS

- Hazmat Inventory
- Hazmat Procedures
- Managing Specific Types of Materials
- Labeling and Safety Data Sheets
- Hazardous Waste Disposal
- Responding to Hazmat Incidents

in other
words

hazardous materials

Dangerous materials (radioactive, flammable, explosive, or poisonous) that would be harmful to people or to the environment if released without taking necessary precautions, as per local, state, and/or federal laws or regulations.

hazardous waste

A term with a specific legal meaning, as determined by the US Environmental Protection Agency (EPA) and the US Department of Transportation (DOT), that applies to certain materials that have been generated as wastes from processes applied to hazardous materials.

KEY CONCEPT

Hazmat Inventory

The first questions to ask about hazardous materials and hazardous waste in your organization are, "What kinds? Where are they? How many are there of each kind?" Good questions. The answers to those should be in your hazmat inventory.

Materials Required in a Hazmat Inventory

Note that your inventory needs to include only hazmat addressed by local, state, and federal law and regulation, including those specified by these agencies:

- Occupational Safety and Health Administration (OSHA)
- Environmental Protection Agency (EPA)
- Department of Transportation (DOT)
- Nuclear Regulatory Commission (NRC)
- Drug Enforcement Administration (DEA)
- Publicly owned treatment works (POTW)

Types of Hazmat

Your inventory may contain many types of hazmat. They typically fall into the categories shown below, as far as Joint Commission Environment of Care (EC) standards are concerned.

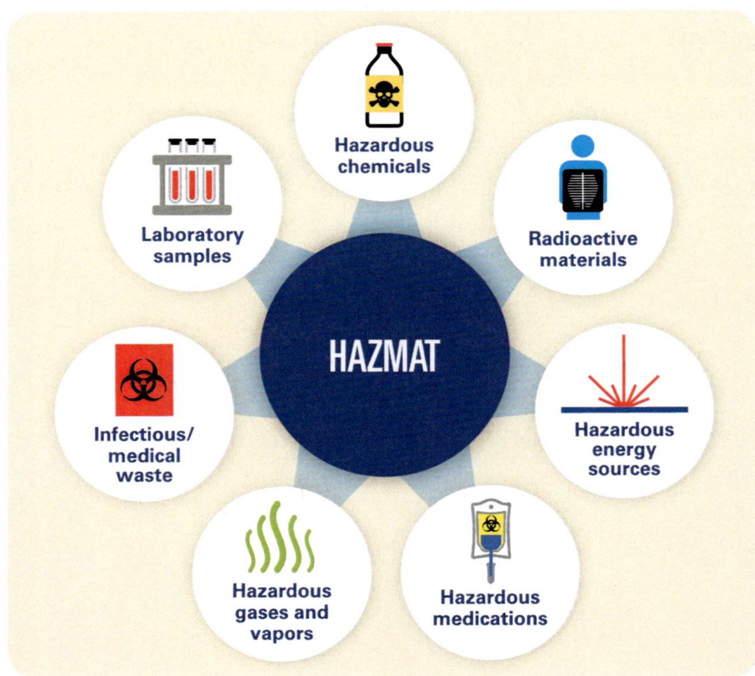

Elements of an Inventory Form

An inventory form can be simple or complex. It may be one sheet of paper or a database divided by category or facility. It all depends on your organization and the hazardous materials and waste you manage. Still, most of them have a lot in common. You should include the inventory location (facility name, department name, room number), inventory taker name, and inventory date, of course. In addition, the following are typically recorded on the forms, for each material—but only a few are *required*:

- **Material name(s):** Complete name on the label of the container. It should match the product name and the name on the safety data sheet (SDS). (For more on the SDS, *see* page 79.) Per OSHA (which EPA references for chemical inventory requirements), the minimal chemical inventory must contain the chemical name and common name as well as synonym names and product/mixture name (if applicable) and percentage of ingredients in product/mixture (if applicable).
- **Manufacturer name:** Name of the company that produced or sold the material. It might also be the name of the vendor who sold it to you. It should match the name on the SDS.
- **SDS on file:** Indicates only that an SDS from the manufacturer is on file. (You need an SDS for any item in this inventory.)
- **CAS/catalog number:** Number assigned by the Chemical Abstracts Service (CAS) or product number in a materials catalog. This is required by the EPA (again, per OSHA). The DOT UN (United Nations) identifier would be an acceptable identifier for this hazardous waste if no CAS number is available.
- **Maximum quantity on hand:** Number of containers on hand at any one time. Knowing this also helps with ordering stock. This isn't required unless the EPA requires you to submit the form (*see* the next section, "EPA submission requirements").
- **Estimated weight/volume:** Total approximate weight/volume of all material on hand at the time of inventory
- **Storage area:** Location of the material in your facility, which should match any location codes on facility site maps

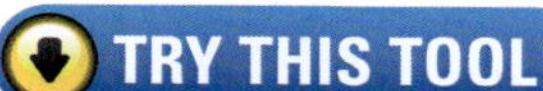

Hazardous Materials Inventory Form
You can use this form for your inventory or incorporate parts of it into your current form, as appropriate.

- **Hazards:** Any health/safety/fire risks, per the SDS
- **PPE:** Any personal protective equipment (PPE) required for managing the material (*see* "Personal Protective Equipment (PPE)" on page 71).
- **Staff training required:** Description of training required to handle the materials (not always on these forms, but helpful)

EPA submission requirements: Note that the EPA requires some organizations to submit their chemical inventory to their State Emergency Response Commission (SERC), Local Emergency Planning Committee (LEPC), and/or local fire department annually by March 1 per Emergency Planning and Community Right-to-Know Act (EPCRA) Sections 311–312 Tier I and Tier II. The facilities required to submit this inventory have chemicals with quantities equal to or greater than the following thresholds (applicable to health care environment)*:

- For extremely hazardous substances (EHSs): 40 CFR part 355 Appendix A and Appendix B, either 500 pounds or the Threshold Planning Quantity (TPQ), whichever is lower
- For all other hazardous chemicals: 10,000 pounds
- Some local governments may require organizations to submit this information to their local fire departments. Contact your local fire department or local fire marshal to verify if this is applicable to your organization.

Definitions: Note that the addition of a column with the definition of Hazardous Chemical (OSHA), Hazardous Material (DOT) or Hazardous Waste (EPA) isn't necessary per Joint Commission standards. But that kind of distinction could be helpful to your organization for your own documentation purposes.

A standardized inventory: If you standardize how you refer to the types of hazardous materials, their locations, and the quantities, it'll help ensure a consistent inventory across your organization and help you to log the materials properly. You might even want to create or find a standardized form, but first check with your state EPA to see if it requires you to use a specific form.

An accurate and complete inventory: Take pains to make sure the hazardous materials inventory is accurate and complete. Inaccuracies can have severe consequences, such as

* Please *see* http://www2.epa.gov/epcra-tier-i-and-tier-ii-reporting/epcra-sections-311-312#covered for more information.

fire, staff injury, patient illness, or even death. Performing the inventory annually will help keep it up to date.

A computerized inventory: Consider making your inventory part of a computerized database—with a backup. It makes updating the inventory much easier. Also, an electronic record of hazardous materials allows staff to quickly and easily access information about a particular hazardous material and its use in the organization.

COLLABORATION: So, who has to actually do the inventory? Well, if you're a facilities director, you may not have to do the inventory yourself, but you may be the one delegating the job. Someone in each department and/or facility in your organization can be trained how to use the form to collect inventory information. Accreditation professionals, think about sitting in on an inventory session to get an overview of the hazardous materials currently used in your organization.

KEY CONCEPT

Hazmat Procedures

Managing hazmat may begin with an inventory, but it doesn't end with inventory, of course. It encompasses the following procedures, all of which may be going on at the same time for any one type of hazardous material in your organization:

- Selecting
- Handling
- Labeling
- Storing
- Transporting
- Using
- Generating
- Monitoring
- Disposing
- Documenting
- Staff training

Contracted services: Many organizations get help with hazmat management because some of the procedures (such as disposing of hazardous waste) require special expertise. If you use contracted services for hazmat, your organization is still ultimately responsible: You have to make sure your vendor meets Joint Commission standards and other laws and regulations. That includes proper licenses, permits, and manifests (*see* the Key Concept "Hazardous Waste Disposal" on page 79).

COLLABORATION: Leaders, part of your responsibility, per Joint Commission standards, is to make sure contract services are meeting expectations. Facilities directors, you may need to solicit performance reports from contractors in hazmat (and other environment of care areas using contract services). Accreditation professionals, you may need to work with facilities directors to advise leaders on what actions to take to improve those services, including providing consultation or training on accreditation requirements to the contractor.

Risk Management of Hazmat Procedures

Another good question to ask about hazardous materials in your organization is, "What kind of risks do they pose?" Remember: Risk management has to be part of your EC management plans (*see* Chapter 2). You can use your inventory as a starting point for this requirement:

- First, make sure each of the hazmat procedures is covered in your relevant EC management plan.
- Then, based on that plan, consider the risks involved in each procedure for *each* type of hazardous material in your inventory, always looking for safer alternatives to hazardous materials.

Selecting New Materials

Your inventory gives you a pretty good picture of which types of hazardous materials are being used in your organization. But you might get requests for more or different products, based on changes in services and other factors, such as cost. When you're selecting new materials, in addition to looking at risks for each hazmat and the procedures involved in its use, evaluate risks such as these:

- Flammability
- Vapors
- Corrosiveness
- Environmental impact
- Special equipment required
- Security required

Limiting authorization: Your organization should also have controls in place to limit the authorization for selecting and purchasing certain products. Not everyone should be able to order cyanide, for instance. Limiting authorization is one of the best ways to maintain control over dangerous materials and reduce risks. One way to do this is to require departments ordering new chemicals to get approval from the EC committee (*see* Chapter 1) or from a hazmat officer before materials management can authorize the purchase.

Personal Protective Equipment (PPE)

Safety glasses, face shields, lead-lined aprons. These are just a few of the many types of personal protective equipment (PPE) health care professionals wear or use on the job to protect themselves from hazardous materials and waste.

Assessing access to hazmat PPE: Health care workers who are required to handle, transport, use, dispose of, or in any way deal with hazardous materials and waste must have access to proper PPE. OSHA requires you to provide a written "certification of hazard assessment." Basically, this documents that you've performed an assessment involving these steps:

Step 1 — Dangers: Identify dangers related to specific hazardous materials.

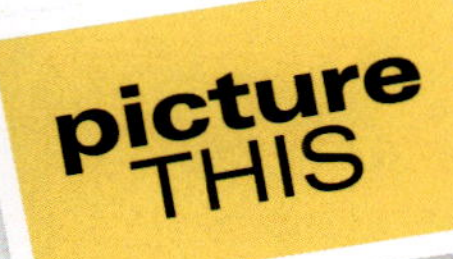

PPE Glove Failure

1. Permeation	2. Penetration	3. Degradation
The glove becomes permeable, allowing a chemical or an agent—including chemotherapy drugs, cytostatic agents, disinfectants, and composite resin materials—to migrate through the glove at a molecular level. 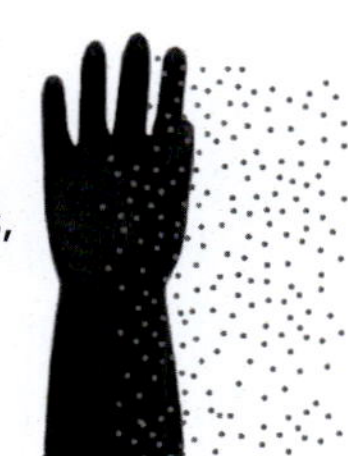	The glove has physical spaces in the material caused by rips, tears, penetrable seams, pinholes, or manufacturing defects that allow the bulk flow-through of a chemical agent or pathogen. 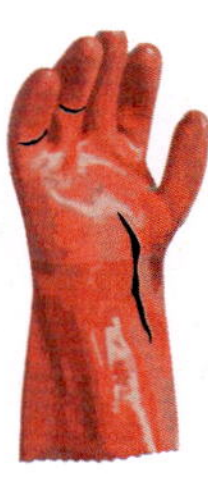	The glove sustains a damaging change in one or more physical properties of the glove material after exposure to a chemical agent, as evidenced by hardening, embrittle-ment, stiffness, cracking, softening, or swelling of the glove. 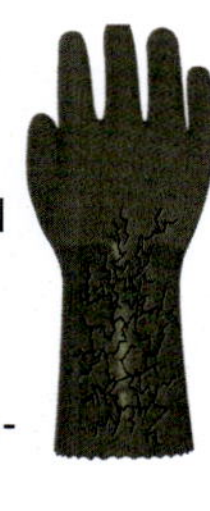

Perhaps the most frequently used PPE of all is gloves. Gloves function as a crucial barrier between hazardous materials and the hands—the body part that most often and easily comes into contact with these materials and spreads them to others. Gloves, however, are susceptible to leaks, permeation, tears, punctures, and deterioration. At some stage, protective gloves will cease to safeguard the wearer because of one (or more) of the three failures, says an OSHA expert.

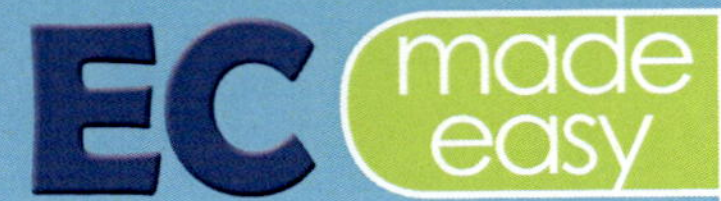

Step 2 — Job functions: Determine specific staff job functions related to those materials.

Step 3 — Appropriate PPE: Assign the appropriate PPE to mitigate hazards for those materials.

Training on hazmat PPE: OSHA also requires your organization to make sure staff know how to use PPE correctly and can demonstrate that before they have contact with any hazardous materials or waste. At a minimum, training should involve the following:

- When PPE is necessary
- What PPE is necessary
- How to properly don, doff, adjust, and wear PPE
- Limitations of the PPE
- Proper care, maintenance, useful life, and disposal of the PPE

KEY CONCEPT

Managing Specific Types of Materials

Caution is fundamental to hazmat, but not standard: Each type of material might need a unique cautionary approach. What follows are a few general issues to consider for select procedures involved in managing specific types of materials.

Hazardous Chemicals

Chemicals of all sorts are used in a health care organization, from cleaning substances in environmental services to various hazardous drugs at nursing stations to reagents of all types in the laboratory to paints, solvents, and fuels in maintenance areas. Other common hazardous chemicals in health care include glutaraldehyde (used in sterilization of medical equipment), formaldehyde (used in labs, histology, and pathology), and waste anesthetic gas (found in surgical areas).

Storing: The storage area for hazardous chemicals should conform to what's required by the SDS forms of the chemicals stored there. And it should be designed to reduce the risks of breakage and spills. It's best to make sure it's secured too, although that's not required.

Handling and using: Adequate ventilation is a primary safe-guard for areas where hazardous chemicals are handled and used—and stored. In some cases, you might need a dedicated exhaust system.

Monitoring: OSHA requires you to monitor staff working with some of these chemicals. This can entail having staff get regular physical examinations to make sure there haven't been any reactions to any exposures.

Radioactive Materials and Hazardous Energy Sources

Radioactive materials are found in radiology, nuclear medicine, and anywhere else in a facility where diagnostic imaging is performed or where patients being treated with radioactive implants are located. Lasers, commonly used in surgical techniques, are an example of a hazardous energy source, because accidental exposure to lasers can cause tissue damage.

Storing and transporting: The NRC requires all health care organizations to store radioactive materials in a secure, locked area and provide a method of supervision for the products. NRC regulations also govern the control of radioactive materials when they're being transported through your facility. The Joint Commission requires compliance with those regulations because NRC is the highest authority having jurisdiction (AHJ) for radioactive materials (*see* Chapter 2).

Monitoring and staff training: As with hazardous chemicals, staff who regularly work with radioactivity need to be monitored routinely for exposure. Using a dosimeter is one way of doing that. Some staff wear dosimeter badges, for example. Make sure they know how to use them correctly and log their read-ings. Staff should also be trained to recognize signs and symptoms of overexposure.

smart questions:

What path do radioactive materials take through your facility? What security measures are in place?

in other words

dosimeter

A device that measures an individual's or an object's exposure to radiated energy.

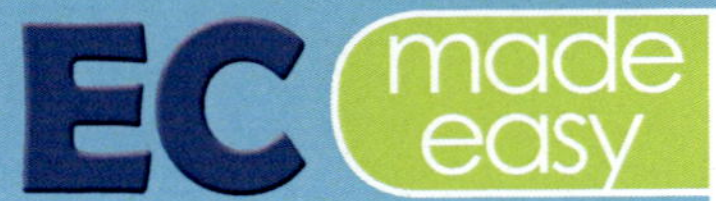

Documenting: With an increase in diagnostic imaging, keeping tabs on the equipment is a priority. Make sure to include all radiation-producing equipment in your medical equipment inventory (*see* Chapter 6). That equipment should be tracked for maintenance and service so any problems can be quickly identified and corrected. And be prepared to immediately remove any recalled models (*see* Chapter 3).

COLLABORATION: Facilities directors, work with your security department in setting up controls for the security of radioactive materials. For example, access to areas containing radioactive material should be restricted to approved personnel only. So, department-level leaders, you need to let facilities directors know exactly who needs access—and whenever that access status for anyone changes. Accreditation professionals, check with any other regulatory staff to see how your state works with the NRC regulations because it varies state to state.

Hazardous Medications

A small percentage of the medications used in the hospital are considered hazardous. The pharmacy should identify these medications and establish a process for other staff, such as nursing, to determine hazardous medications from nonhazardous medications. Pharmacy should review hazardous drugs to determine proper personal protective equipment and disposal requirements.

Some of the most toxic medications, chemotherapeutic agents, are intended to destroy malignant cells but can have the same effect on healthy cells. That's why staff should use extreme care when working with these agents, including disposal of their packaging.

Handling and using: When drugs are administered, the tubing or port connections may not be properly secured, which can cause accidents to occur. Another reason why use of PPE is so critical. It's also important for those administering the drugs to know proper spill cleanup procedures.

Transporting and storing: Hazardous drugs can cause environmental contamination in a variety of ways. Drug containers may be damaged when shipped, resulting in spills or leakage into other materials—both in transport and in storage after transport. The DOT requires special containers to be used for transportation of hazardous medication waste.

Disposing and staff training: Whether it's in the pharmacy, an inpatient oncology unit, or outpatient infusion area, someone is going to have to dispose of chemo drug packaging. Unlike disposal of some other types of hazardous materials, it might be clinical staff who dispose of the packaging, so training is paramount. Yellow containers are typically used for empty vials, intravenous (IV) bags and tubing, and personal protective equipment used to administer chemotherapy to patients. Black containers are often used to dispose of vials still containing chemotherapy drugs and certain other hazardous medication disposal. Talk to pharmacy to understand the different colors of containers used for hazardous drug disposal.

Hazardous Gases and Vapors

Medical gases and vapors can be some of the most dangerous hazardous materials in your facility—and not just because some are invisible *and* flammable. In addition to the safety measures outlined in Chapter 3 for labeling and storing full and empty medical gas cylinders, consider the risk issues described below.

Storing and staff training: Although not required by law or regulation, it's a good idea to keep medical gas cylinders secured from unauthorized access—while making sure they're accessible to staff. In this case, secure storage is also about preventing cylinders from becoming damaged or ruptured, per NFPA regulation. Make sure major tank repairs are completed by qualified staff, per Joint Commission Human Resources (HR) standards.

Using: Surgical procedures that use a laser unit can produce a smoke byproduct that may contain toxic gases and vapors. Smoke evacuators can help remove surgical smoke.

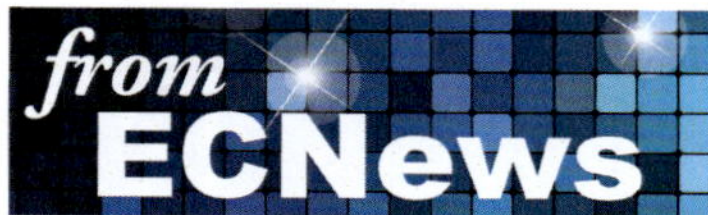

Hazardous Drugs
Health care workers are typically exposed to the remnants of harmful agents via contaminated clothing, airborne particles, spills, needlestick injuries, and human waste. It is believed that absorption of hazardous drugs most commonly occurs through contact between unprotected skin and contaminated surfaces.

A higher incidence of exposure is likely where hazardous drugs are most commonly handled, including areas where medication mixing, infusion, disposal, spill management, and waste containment occur.

Consider that hazardous residue on the surfaces of contaminated drug vials can be transferred via hospital staff who receive, store, and take inventory of the substance. Even if they wear gloves, the debris can transfer to other surfaces that fellow workers can come into contact with. Even trace remnants of some drugs can dry, vaporize, become airborne, and be inhaled.

—excerpted from
"Menacing Meds: How to Safely Manage Hazardous Drugs in the Health Care Environment,"
Environment of Care® News,
March 2014

Monitoring: Laws and regulations require frequent monitoring of gases and vapors, including staying within acceptable ranges. It's especially important to monitor and manage the nonflammable medical gases stored in patient care areas.

Infectious/Medical Waste

Regulated medical waste, biohazardous waste, biomedical waste, infectious/medical waste. Whatever you call it, this waste material needs to be properly handled at all times to prevent spread of infection:

- When it's generated
- When it's labeled
- When it's transported
- When it's disposed of

In the Joint Commission standards, infectious/medical waste is technically covered by the Infection Prevention and Control (IC) standards. But EC and IC standards both require keeping the physical environment clean and clear of infection.

Disposing: Preventing infection during *use* of sharps (needles and other sharp instruments) was addressed in Chapter 3. Disposing of them *after use* can create risks of its own. Proper use of sharps disposal containers can help reduce those risks (*see* the sidebar "Reducing Sharps Infection Risks During Disposal" below). Reminders on the correct use of biohazardous or red bags reduces risks too—in addition to keeping down expenses incurred when the bags are used for nonhazardous waste.

in other words

sharps

Medical instruments (such as scalpels or hypodermic needles) that are sharp or may produce sharp pieces by shattering.

biohazardous or red bag

A plastic bag that is either red in color or is labeled with a biohazard symbol used by health care facilities for the disposal of "non-sharp" and potentially infectious biohazardous waste.

Reducing Sharps Infection Risks During Disposal

Consider using these approaches to reduce infectious/medical waste risks when disposing of sharps in sharps containers:

- Maintain containers upright throughout use.
- Replace them routinely to prevent breaking from wear and tear.
- Monitor the "full-line" to make sure containers are not overfilled.
- Locate them close to where sharps are used.
- Place containers ergonomically to avoid injuries from awkward angles of access.
- Mount or place containers in stands to avoid spillage.

- Label the containers with the universal biohazard symbol or color-code them red.
- Lock (if a mobile cart is used) containers to prevent unintentional access or removal.
- Follow all applicable state regulations regarding sharps containers.
- Place the containers away from easy access by patients and visitors (especially in exam rooms where patients might bring their children).

Labeling and Safety Data Sheets

Labels can save lives. They can allow staff to quickly identify hazardous materials and the level of risk the materials may pose. But they need to be clear to everyone. So you should have a labeling system that all staff understand and recognize.

Hazmat Labeling

Hazmat labeling is addressed in the Joint Commission standards, but it's primarily OSHA's Hazard Communication Standard (HCS) that drives your hazmat label requirements. And labels are just the first part of a series of new requirements from the revised HCS to be implemented in the coming years.

HCS HazCom Labels: OSHA requires the following elements on all hazardous chemical labels, known as the HCS HazCom Labels:
- **Product identifier:** Typically a code and product name
- **Supplier identification:** Contact information for the supplier
- **Hazard pictograms:** Standardized, universal symbols; selection determined by chemical hazard classification
- **Signal word:** A single warning word, such as *Danger*
- **Hazard statement(s):** Warnings about health hazards
- **Precautionary statement(s):** Warnings about handling or use

NFPA's labeling system: If you have a chemical or fire emergency, responders need to know—at a glance—the dangers of chemicals present in your facility. To help protect those emergency workers, the NFPA requires a specific labeling system, per NFPA 704, *Standard System for the Identification of the Hazards of Materials for Emergency Response*. The system consists of colors (blue, red, yellow, and white) and numbers on a diamond-shaped label. They indicate hazard ratings for the following for any hazardous materials:
- Health
- Flammability
- Instability
- Special hazards

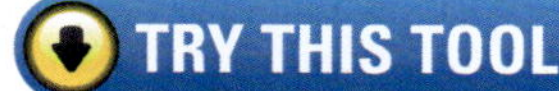

TRY THIS TOOL

OSHA QuickCard™: Hazard Communication Standard Labels
This QuickCard™ by OSHA provides an example of what a hazardous materials label should look like.

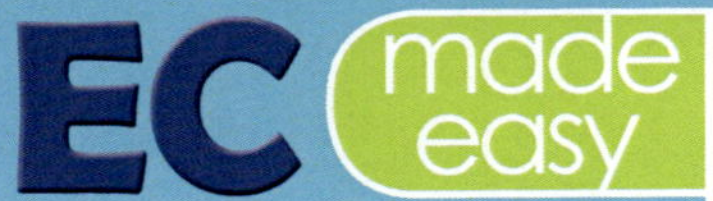

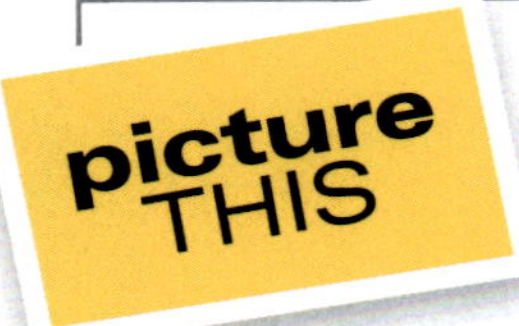

OSHA Hazardous Materials Pictograms

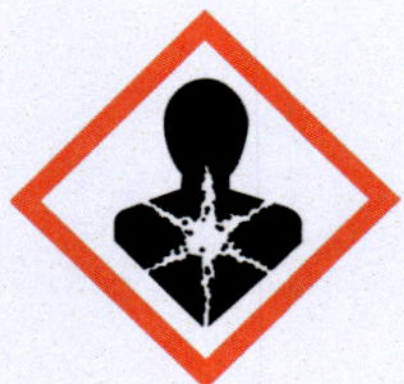

Health Hazard:
Carcinogen, Mutagenicity,
Reproductive Toxicity,
Respiratory Sensitizer, Target
Organ Toxicity,
Aspiration Toxicity

Flame:
Flammables, Pyrophorics,
Self-Heating, Emits
Flammable Gas, Self-Reactives,
Organic Peroxides

Exclamation Mark:
Irritant (skin and eye), Skin
Sensitizer, Acute Toxicity
(harmful), Narcotic Effects,
Respiratory Tract Irritant,
Hazardous to Ozone Layer
(Non-Mandatory)

Gas Cylinder:
Gases Under Pressure

Corrosion:
Skin Corrosion/Burns, Eye
Damage, Corrosive to Metals

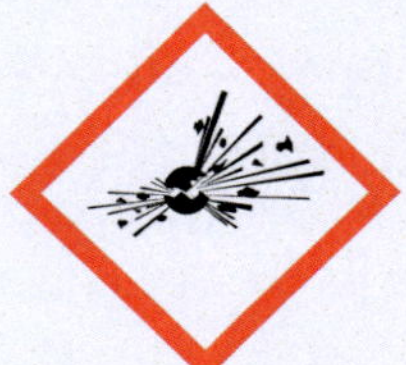

Exploding Bomb:
Explosives, Self-Reactives,
Organic Peroxides

Flame Over Circle:
Oxidizers

Environment (Non-Mandatory):
Aquatic Toxicity

Skull and Crossbones:
Acute Toxicity (fatal or toxic)

OSHA's revised HCS includes requirements for hazard pictograms pictured here. Each pictogram represents particular types of hazards, as shown. Which pictogram you use on a label is determined by OSHA's chemical hazard classification. These classifications are listed for each pictogram. Directions for creating the labels are available on the OSHA website.

In many organizations, contracted vendors might supply hazardous materials, such as tanks of liquid oxygen. They're supposed to supply the tanks already marked with the NFPA diamond. But your organization needs to be sure the tanks are marked correctly.

Safety Data Sheets

Safety data sheets (SDSs) are some of the most important documents in your organization. Formerly called material safety data sheets, their purpose is to provide detailed information about hazardous materials. OSHA's revised HCS requires the following for SDSs:

- **Format of SDSs:** All SDSs must use OSHA's 16-section uniform SDS format.
- **Provision of SDSs:** Manufacturers and vendors of hazardous chemicals are required by law to provide purchasers with an SDS for each chemical.
- **SDSs in your facility:** You must have an SDS for each hazardous chemical stored or used at your facility, per your hazmat inventory. Also, you must keep relevant SDSs in work areas where the chemicals are stored. And, perhaps most importantly, you must make all of them easily available to staff, preferably in a central location.

Hazardous Waste Disposal

Unlike hazardous materials, hazardous waste can't do anyone any good. It must be disposed of properly—which means very carefully. That's why several federal regulatory agencies oversee hazardous waste disposal processes. OSHA, the EPA, and the DOT require a host of permits and licenses for disposal services and activities, and all must be maintained and kept current.

Hazardous Waste Manifest System

You're responsible, as a hazardous waste generator, for determining your generator status by types and volumes of hazardous waste—and for meeting all regulatory requirements associated with that status.

---

in other words

safety data sheet (SDS)
A sheet provided by the manufacturer that includes details about a substance's hazards. Employers must make sure that SDSs (formerly known as material safety data sheets) are readily accessible to employees.

smart questions:
Where do you have all the SDSs filed for staff to access?

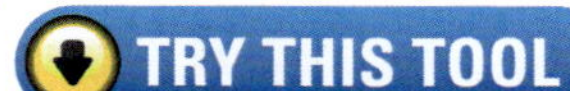

Hazardous Waste Storage Inspection Checklist
Make sure your hazardous waste storage areas are safe by using this checklist.

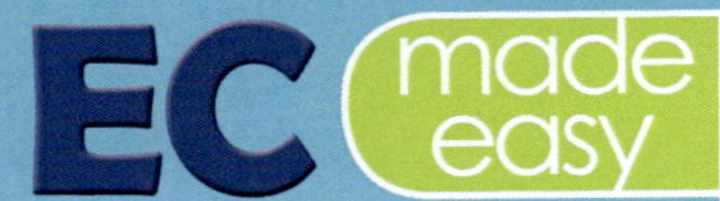

The EPA and DOT regulate the hazardous waste manifest system. This system is a set of training, labeling, forms, reports, and procedures for tracking hazardous waste from where it's generated to the off-site waste management facility where it's stored, treated, or disposed of. It's also used when transporting infectious substances for further lab analysis or infections medical waste. The part of the system most important to you is the EPA's Uniform Hazardous Waste Manifest. Basically, if you're going on a public road with hazardous substances, you're going to need this manifest.

Uniform Hazardous Waste Manifest: This form, required by the EPA and the DOT, is one of various hazmat manifests you may need, depending on your city and state. It documents the type and quantity of hazardous waste you're sending out for disposal. Here are a few things you need to know:

- **One per shipment:** The DOT requires one of these manifests for every shipment of hazardous substances from your facility.
- **Multiple copies:** The form provides multiple copies. All parties (both generator and shipper) sign the form and keep a copy for themselves as documentation. You'll get a signed copy of the manifest back from the waste hauler. That provides a record of proper disposal.
- **Staff training:** The manifests are complex. The DOT requires staff training for completing them.
- **Form source:** You have to use the EPA form. You can get it from any source approved by the EPA Manifest Registry to print and distribute the form, such as your state EPA.
- **State requirements:** Your state might have additional requirements related to the form.

COLLABORATION: Your health care organization's hazardous materials and waste program must comply with all federal, state, and local laws and regulations. The Joint Commission defers to these, so facilities directors and accreditation professionals, you should know what they are. And accreditation professionals, you'll want to pay particular attention to hazardous materials disposal, because some organizations have received stiff penalties for noncompliance. Hazardous waste generator status is determined by types and volumes of

in other words

hazmat manifest

A form issued by governmental agencies that's used to track hazardous waste as it travels from where it's generated to the waste management facility that will store, treat, or dispose of it.

smart questions:

What manifests are required by your state and city for disposal of hazardous waste from your facility?

hazardous waste generated. Organizations are responsible for determining their generator status and meeting all regulatory requirements associated with it.

The Risks of Disposal

When disposing of hazardous materials and waste, it's vital that all materials be handled in a way that minimizes risks. You also need to implement processes that allow you to monitor and easily report any risks. To do that, focus on the following:

- **Separation:** Keep hazardous waste storage and processing areas separate from sterile areas and clean supplies.
- **Classification:** Separate hazardous waste by type and keep it away from ordinary trash.
- **Transport:** Establish a minimal travel distance between the site of final use and a protected disposal unit.
- **Documentation:** Track the waste collection and handling processes to allow for continuous monitoring and evaluation of your efforts and to better comply with regulations.
- **Contractor:** If you use a contractor, select a reputable and experienced one and evaluate the effectiveness on an ongoing basis.

For more information on OSHA regulations and consultation programs for disposing of hazardous waste in your state, visit the Healthcare Environmental Resource Center (HERC) website.

KEY CONCEPT

Responding to Hazmat Incidents

If there's a hazardous material spill, you have to act fast. The safety of patients, staff, and visitors in your health care facility is at stake. All staff should know how to respond to spills, accidents, inhalation, and personal contact involving hazardous materials and waste.

Using the Hazmat Inventory and the SDSs

The first step in responding to a spill is knowing which chemicals and other hazardous materials could present a problem. This provides another instance in which your inventory is invaluable. You'll know the types, quantities, and locations of hazardous materials. And you'll have access to the SDSs, so you'll also know details about the hazards associated with each material.

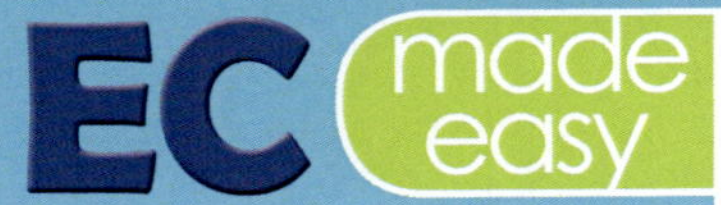

Drenching Facilities

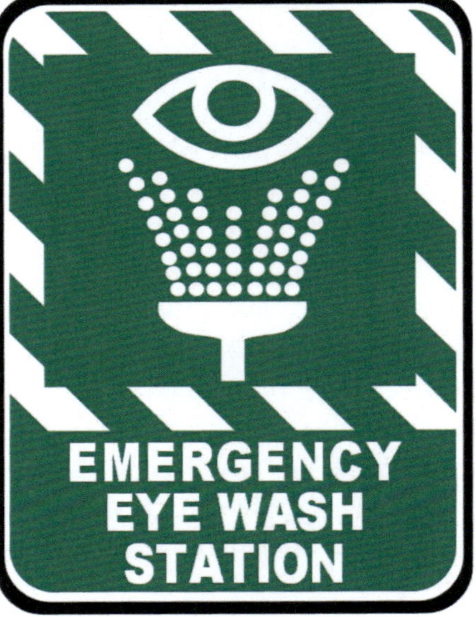

If your staff come in contact with corrosives on the job, they need access to drenching facilities. Drenching facilities include eyewash or eye/face wash stations and showers. What you need depends on the extent of the exposure and the type of hazardous material. For hazardous chemicals, OSHA requires that you have a full-drench shower available. OSHA defers to the American National Standards Institute (ANSI) for the specific requirements for drenching equipment. ANSI developed a standard specifically for eyewashes and showers. It requires you to have an emergency eyewash and shower on the same level as the hazard, unobstructed access, and within 10 seconds from the hazard area. It also addresses training staff in using them correctly.

Hazmat Spill Response Procedures

Joint Commission standards also require you to have written procedures that detail the steps involved in response to a hazmat spill. This might involve identifying specific individuals or a team to respond to all or certain types of spills. These steps should include the following:

- Precautionary tactics
- PPE to use following a spill
- Containment of a spill (preventing it from spreading)
- Proper cleanup and disposal of spilled materials
  (*see* the sidebar "Hazmat Spill Kit" below)

Hazmat Spill Kit

You should put spill control kits (or spill kits) in all areas involving use of hazardous materials that could spill.

Spill Kit Contents
- Spill cleanup instructions
- Warning signs to post
- Personal protective equipment (PPE)
- Absorbent sheets/spill pads
- Disposable towels
- Thick sealable plastic waste disposal bags and ties (two large and several small)
- A disposable scoop
- Sharps container for glass fragments

Using a Spill Kit
Before making use of a spill kit, inform the appropriate person in your area and call for help, if necessary. Then open the spill kit and follow the instructions. Usually, they follow these basic steps:

➤ **Step 1:** Read the spill kit instructions.

➤ **Step 2:** Block access to the spill by posting the warning signs in the kit.

➤ **Step 3:** Don the PPE (including two pairs of gloves); separate the towels, sheets, pads, and bags; and prepare two large bags to hold the used spill material.

➤ **Step 4:** Blanket any spilled powder with a wet towel before picking it up and gather any glass fragments into the sharps container.

➤ **Step 5:** Place absorbent materials on a liquid spill; when saturated, put them in the small sealable bags. When each bag is full, seal it and place it into the large bag.

➤ **Step 6:** After the spill is contained, use detergent to wash the area; rinse the area with water three times. Absorb all wash/rinse water and contain it in a small bag.

➤ **Step 7:** Place all used supplies in the large bag and tie it off. Place that bag, along with all PPE (except inner gloves), into a second large bag. Seal that bag, insert it into a container labeled as hazardous waste, and seal it. Set the container aside to be picked up later by appropriate staff.

➤ **Step 8:** Remove inner gloves and seal them in a small bag, which should be placed into another hazardous waste container. Wash hands and arms thoroughly with soap and warm water.

➤ **Step 9:** Record the spill details, complete an incident report/exposure form, and report the spill to the emergency department to be evaluated for adverse health effects.

Source: National Institute for Occupational Safety and Health (NIOSH)

Outside help: In many cases your organization may be able to handle a spill on its own. But depending on the size of the spill and the type of hazardous material, you may need to contact an outside resource. Your local fire department, for example, might be better equipped to handle large incidents.

Hazmat spill training: After procedures are set, get everyone trained. Training should be based on the most current information about the products. That information comes from several sources, which you should gather on an ongoing basis:

- **Primary sources:** Primary data sources include the following:
  - Manufacturers
  - Suppliers
  - Regulatory agencies
  - Environmental rounds or tours
  - The materials management department
- **Other sources:** Other sources of information may include the National Institute for Occupational Safety and Health (NIOSH), part of the US Centers for Disease Control and Prevention (CDC), or your organization's infection control and safety programs.

TOOLS OF THE TRADE

- Hazardous Materials Inventory Form
- Dosimeter Log
- OSHA QuickCard™: Hazard Communication Standard Labels
- Hazardous Waste Storage Inspection Checklist

CHAPTER 6

CHAPTER 6

Medical Equipment and Utility Systems

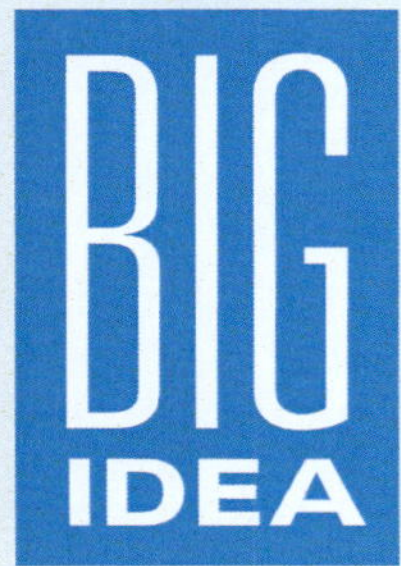

Very few patient care processes can take place without medical equipment. And if it malfunctions, it can cause health complications, injury, or even death. A similar functional focus is necessary for utility systems that provide clean water, appropriate pressure relationships for sterile and isolated areas, heating and cooling, and other essential elements that effect the health care environment on a daily basis. Maintenance and monitoring are a constant aspect of managing these vital components of health care. As medical equipment and utility systems become more advanced, so too must the management programs in your facility.

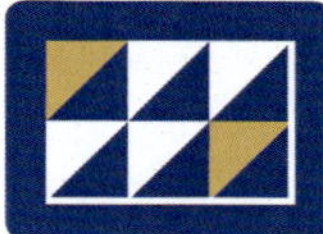

THE MANUAL

Following are the relevant Joint Commission *Comprehensive Accreditation Manual (CAM)* chapters:

- Environment of Care (EC)
- Leadership (LD)
- Infection Prevention and Control (IC)

KEY CONCEPTS

- Medical Equipment: Managing the Program
- Medical Equipment: Inventory
- Medical Equipment: Maintenance
- Medical Equipment: Responding to Failures
- Equipment Management (EQ)
- Utility Systems: Managing the Program
- Utility Systems: Inventory of Operating Components
- Utility Systems: Maintenance
- Utility Systems: Infection Control
- Utility Systems: Piped Medical Gas
- Utility Systems: Emergency Power Supply System
- Utility Systems: Responding to Failures

Chapter Key Concepts	AHC	BHC	CAH	HAP	LAB	NCC	OBS	OME
Medical Equipment								
• Managing the Program	✖		✖	✖	✖		✖	
• Inventory	✖		✖	✖	✖			
• Maintenance	✖		✖	✖	✖	✖	✖	
• Responding to Failures	✖		✖	✖		✖	✖	
• Equipment Management (EQ)								✖
Utility Systems								
• Managing the Program	✖	✖	✖	✖	✖	✖	✖	✖
• Inventory of Operating Components			✖	✖	✖			
• Maintenance	✖	✖	✖	✖	✖	✖	✖	✖
• Infection Control	✖		✖	✖	✖	✖	✖	
• Piped Medical Gas	✖		✖	✖		✖		
• Emergency Power Supply System	✖	✖	✖	✖	✖	✖	✖	✖
• Responding to Failures	✖	✖	✖	✖	✖	✖	✖	✖

AHC—Ambulatory Health Care; BHC—Behavioral Health Care; CAH—Critical Access Hospital; HAP—Hospital; LAB—Laboratory and Point-of-Care Testing; NCC—Nursing Care Centers; OBS—Office-Based Surgery; OME—Home Care.

Joint Commission Environment of Care (EC) standards require organizations to manage risk associated with medical equipment and utilities and to inspect, test, and maintain them to keep them from failing. This varies by accreditation program setting. Use the chart above to see which sections of this chapter apply to your accreditation setting.

in other words

medical equipment

Fixed or portable equipment used in any stage of patient care; not the same as *medical devices* (any instrument, apparatus, implant, in vitro reagent, or similar or related article that is used to diagnose, prevent, or treat disease or other conditions) or *medical supplies*.

* For laboratory settings, this is in regard to laboratory equipment.

KEY CONCEPT

Medical Equipment: Managing the Program

For Ambulatory Health Care, Critical Access Hospitals, Hospitals, Laboratory, and Office-Based Surgery*

An effective medical equipment management program depends on a good EC management plan that incorporates thorough risk assessments (*see* Chapter 2). It also depends on good judgment and experience with various types of medical equipment.

Types of Medical Equipment

Your program may use various types of medical equipment, such as the following:

- **Monitoring equipment:** For recording and tracking patient conditions (such as bedside monitors and telemetry monitors)
- **Treatment equipment:** For direct patient care (lasers, diathermy machines)
- **Diagnostic equipment:** For analysis and diagnosis (laboratory analyzers, radiology equipment, endoscopes)
- **Patient support equipment:** For supporting patient health during diagnosis and treatment (beds, lifts)
- **Life-support equipment:** For sustaining life (ventilators, anesthesia machines, heart-lung bypass machines, defibrillators)
- **Laboratory equipment:** For use in diagnosing disease or other conditions

High-risk medical equipment: Whatever type of medical equipment you have, some of it is bound to be classed as *high risk*. What makes it high risk? If it fails, patients or staff may suffer serious injury or even death. Clearly, all life-support equipment is high risk. So is certain equipment used in surgery (robotics). Operating components of your facility's utility systems that pose serious injury or death risks if they fail are also considered high-risk equipment.

What medical equipment must be managed: Your organization's medical equipment management program should address all medical equipment in your facilities regardless of ownership. This includes the following:

- Equipment directly monitored by an in-house clinical engineering department
- Leased equipment
- Patient-owned equipment brought into your facility

Who manages the equipment: Ideally, equipment management is a joint effort between clinical engineering and clinical care services. To have a successful partnership, everyone involved should understand the following about every piece of equipment:

- How it operates
- How it's used in the care environment
- How it's maintained (including validation of inspection)

in other words

life-support equipment

Any medical equipment with the purpose of sustaining life. If it fails to perform its primary function (when used according to the manufacturer's instructions and clinical protocol), that failure will lead to patient death unless there's immediate intervention.

high-risk equipment

Any medical equipment or operating components of utility systems that may result in serious injury or death to patients or staff if it fails. High-risk medical equipment includes life-support equipment. The term is equivalent to the US Centers for Medicare & Medicaid Services (CMS) term *critical equipment.*

COLLABORATION: Effective medical equipment management also depends on integrating processes, coordinating communication, and creating an exchange of information between the groups involved. That requires collaboration. Clinical engineers typically maintain medical equipment. But it's the clinical nursing staff who use it most frequently, so they'll be the first to identify potential problems. Nursing leaders, you need to get that feedback from nursing staff and promptly pass it on to the engineers. Environmental services staff may be asked to clean and, sometimes, store the equipment. Make sure they have the skill, product, and space. Accreditation professionals and facilities directors, you can help support that collaboration. How? By serving as a liaison via membership on the EC committee and clinical committees focused on safety.

Selecting Medical Equipment

Most medical equipment in your organization probably has broad usage. But there may be some equipment used exclusively by certain individuals or departments. Following are guidelines on selecting medical equipment.

Interdisciplinary input: Whenever you select any medical equipment, it's a best practice to get input from those who operate and maintain the equipment. This is a Joint Commission requirement for hospitals and critical access hospitals, and for laboratories when selecting new laboratory equipment. One of the best ways to do this is to establish a selection process involving an interdisciplinary team. That way, you can choose equipment that meets everyone's needs and is compatible with existing equipment.

Evaluating equipment: Requests for medical equipment typically originate in the department where it'll be used. After the request has been made to the selection/procurement team, the team should evaluate the equipment before issuing a purchase order. Here are some things for the team to consider:

- **Purpose and scope:** How the equipment is intended to be used, including the extent of its application in your organization
- **Human factors:** How people will use the equipment, in terms of human factors. For example, if users are familiar with devices using calculator-style keypads, would

unintentional errors occur if new devices use the keypad layout of a cellphone?

- **Maintenance requirements:** The demands of documentation, needs for repair services, and availability of parts. Servicing equipment often requires tools that simulate use conditions. A typical acquisition strategy is to include in the purchase agreement test protocols and equipment.
- **Cleaning requirements:** How the equipment will be cleaned, sterilized, or disinfected, including how facilities or environmental services staff need to be trained to do so.
- **Training requirements:** Who will need what kind of training as well as how that training will be provided. Those who use, maintain, and repair the equipment all need training on operations and protocols. That training is often offered by the manufacturer.
- **Inventory:** If the new piece of equipment needs to be part of your inventory

KEY CONCEPT

Medical Equipment: Inventory

For Ambulatory Health Care, Critical Access Hospitals, Hospitals, and Laboratory*

For deemed status: *See* the sidebar "Medical Equipment and Utility Systems: Inventory and Maintenance for Deemed-Status Hospitals and Critical Access Hospitals" on page 90 for additional or different requirements related to information in this key concept section.

The Joint Commission EC standards require an organization to maintain a written inventory of its medical equipment. Unless your organization is a deemed-status hospital or a critical access hospital, you can choose to take one of two approved approaches[†]:

- **All equipment:** Inventory every item of medical equipment.

OR

- **Selected equipment:** Inventory selected equipment, categorized by risk.

smart questions:

Where is the medical equipment inventory and who is responsible for keeping it up to date?

* For laboratory settings, this is in regard to laboratory equipment.

† Laboratories are required to maintain an inventory of laboratory equipment and equipment incident history.

Medical Equipment and Utility Systems: Inventory and Maintenance for Deemed-Status Hospitals and Critical Access Hospitals

The Joint Commission standards for medical equipment and utility components align with the US Centers for Medicare & Medicaid Services (CMS) requirements for deemed-status hospitals and critical access hospitals (*see* Chapter 1).

The way deemed-status organizations must manage medical equipment and operating components of utility systems inventory and maintenance differs, in some respects, from other, non-deemed accreditation programs. If your organization is a hospital or critical access hospital seeking deemed status, you must do the following for those items:

- **Inventory items:** Include all medical equipment and operating components of utility systems in your inventories (*see* pages 89 and 105).
- **Maintenance activities and frequencies:** Identify maintenance activities and frequencies for all medical equipment and operating components of utility systems on the inventory (*see* pages 92 and 106). This can be done by equipment class.
- **Performance checks:** Do performance checks before initial use (*see* page 94) *and also after major repairs or upgrades* of medical equipment and operating components of utility systems on the inventory. Because repairs and upgrades can sometimes fundamentally change performance, engaging in safety, operational, and functional checks at this time ensures that the equipment or component is in working order and is able to support strong and safe patient care.
- **Nuclear medicine equipment:** Inspect, test, and calibrate nuclear medicine equipment every 12 months and document it (in addition to the requirements for sterilizers and hemodialysis and water testing equipment outlined on page 94).
- **Manufacturers' recommendations:** Use manufacturers' recommendations for maintenance activities and frequencies for these types of medical equipment and operating components of utility systems (*see* page 94):
  - Medical laser devices
  - Imaging and radiologic equipment: This might be for diagnostic or therapeutic purposes.
  - Medical equipment and operating components of utility systems subject to federal or state law or CMS: In this case, organizations may choose to follow manufacturers' recommendations or an approach that establishes more stringent maintenance requirements.
  - New medical equipment or operating components of utility systems that don't have sufficient maintenance history to support use of alternative equipment maintenance (AEM) strategies (*see* the sidebar "AEM Program" on page 95): Sufficient maintenance history in this context includes records provided by the hospital's contractors, information made public by nationally recognized sources, and records of the hospital's experience over time.
- **AEM selections:** Follow these stipulations when selecting medical equipment and operating components of utility systems for an AEM program:
  - Qualified individual: Ensure that only a qualified individual makes those decisions, based on written criteria that take into account the following factors for the item:
    - How it's used
    - What might happen if it fails
    - What alternatives exist if it fails
    - What the incident history is for this equipment or similar equipment
    - What kind of maintenance is required
  - Identified on the inventory: The inventory must identify medical equipment and operating components of utility systems that are part of an AEM program.

Evaluating Medical Equipment Risks

If you decide (and are permitted) to inventory only selected medical equipment, it's a best practice to develop a "risk rank." This can help you determine which equipment should be in your inventory: The higher the risk rank, the more likely the item should be in the inventory. You might also consider using a standardized risk assessment process.

Risk criteria: Consider these risk criteria as you make your decisions:

- **Function:** What's the equipment supposed to do?
- **Physical risk:** What level of risk—to patients and staff— is associated with its use? What might happen if it fails?
- **Incident history:** How many adverse events have involved this equipment? What level of severity is each event?
- **Maintenance requirements:** What's involved in making sure the equipment is always functioning properly? If it requires preventive maintenance (*see* page 94) and doesn't have that, what might happen?
- **Operation and cleaning:** Who cleans the equipment (clinical staff or environmental services)? And who ensures that instructions for use are followed?
- **Regulations and requirements:** Are there state or other accreditation requirements that influence whether this item needs to be in your inventory?

Identifying High-Risk Medical Equipment

You should include all high-risk medical equipment in your inventory and identify it as high risk (you're required to do that if your organization is a hospital or critical access hospital). You might decide to make the identifier more clear and unique by use of a color code or a symbol. Or you might decide to identify the items by putting them into a special section of your inventory identified as a high-risk equipment section.

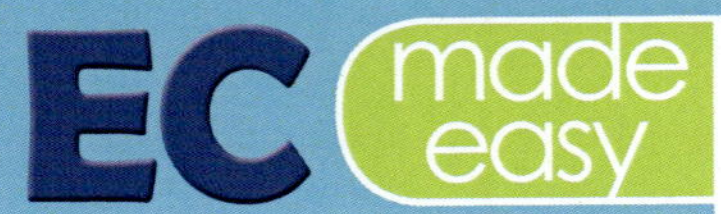

KEY CONCEPT

Medical Equipment: Maintenance

For Ambulatory Health Care, Critical Access Hospitals, Hospitals, Laboratory, Nursing Care Centers, and Office-Based Surgery*

For deemed status: *See* the sidebar "Medical Equipment and Utility Systems: Inventory and Maintenance for Deemed-Status Hospitals and Critical Access Hospitals" on page 90 for additional or different requirements related to information in this key concept section.

Your inventory is done. Now it's time to determine the inspecting, testing, and maintenance involved in making sure all the equipment in the inventory does what it's supposed to do. And then, of course, you have to perform those activities—and perform them on time. You also need to document those activities within an inventory, policy, procedure, work order, or other format.

Activities and Frequencies

The activities of inspecting, testing, and maintaining equipment are generally referred to by the overarching concept of *maintenance activities, preventive maintenance*, or just *maintenance*. Exactly when you need to perform those activities is based on accepted or required frequencies (time intervals). Pretty basic, right? Well, there are some wrinkles—and some special cases.

Joint Commission time definitions: Some Joint Commission standards specify time frequencies, in accord with Joint Commission official time definitions. You're expected to know what those are, and to follow them.

All items on your inventory: Per the standards, all medical equipment on your inventory should be inspected, tested, and maintained as part of your medical equipment management plan. That's one reason why it's so important that you carefully evaluate (if you have that choice) what does and what doesn't need to be on your inventory. Be sure to include equipment

---

Medical Equipment and Utility Systems: Documentation Checklist
Use this checklist to document maintenance of medical equipment and utilities.

* For laboratory settings, this is in regard to laboratory equipment.

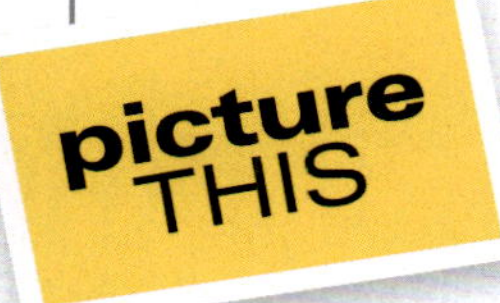

Joint Commission Official Time Definitions

Many standards, including those related to equipment maintenance activities, include designations of time. The following are the Joint Commission official time definitions.

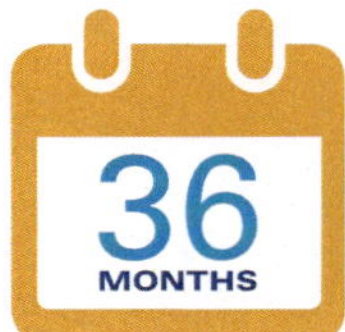

Triennially/every 36 months/every 3 years =
36 months from the date of the last event,
plus or minus 45 days

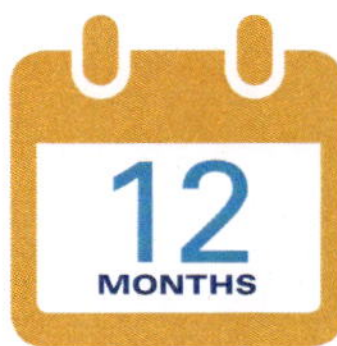

Annually/every 12 months/once a year/every year =
1 year from the date of the last event,
plus or minus 30 days

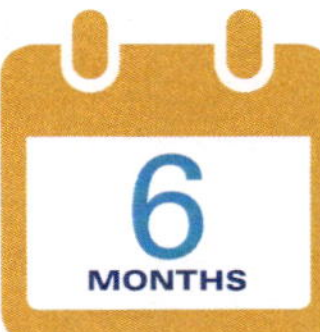

Every 6 months =
6 months from the date of the last event,
plus or minus 20 days

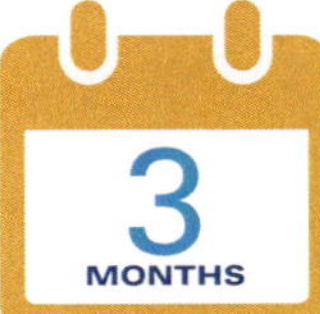

Quarterly/every quarter =
Every three months, plus or minus 10 days

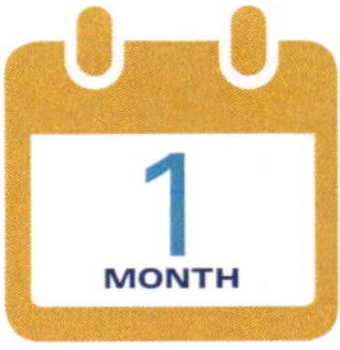

Monthly/30-day intervals/every month =
12 times a year, once per month

Every week =
Once per week

such as sterilizers, hemodialysis and water testing equipment, and laboratory equipment in your medical equipment management plan.

Before first use: To be safe, before anyone in your organization uses any piece of medical equipment brought into your organization for the first time, you're required to conduct performance checks. Check it for safety, operation, and functionality. This applies to the following:

- New equipment
- Leased or rented equipment
- Equipment for trial or demonstration
- Patient-owned equipment

High-risk medical equipment: All high-risk medical equipment must be inspected, tested, and maintained as well. Organizations that elect the Joint Commission Behavioral Health Home option are also required to inspect, test, and maintain medical equipment, although in that case, it doesn't include equipment owned by individuals served or other organizations.

Sterilizers: The Joint Commission has specific requirements for the performance testing and maintenance of all sterilizers. Departments such as sterile processing, laboratory, or surgery areas are typically responsible for doing that and keeping documentation on it.

Hemodialysis and water testing: In addition, maintenance and documentation is required for equipment used in hemodialysis (for kidney failure), as well as chemical and biological testing of water. Proper tests must be performed, and access to any testing documentation should be available even if dialysis is done on a contract basis. This isn't required for laboratory or office-based surgery settings.

Laboratory equipment: Laboratories have quite a few special requirements for equipment maintenance, so check your appropriate manual for those.

Medical Equipment Maintenance Methods

Methods of maintenance may vary. Normally, the method is based on what's appropriate for a particular type of equipment. The Joint Commission understands that. You can pick one of two approved maintenance approaches for any item of medical equipment:

- **Manufacturers' strategies:** Use strategies outlined in the manufacturers' recommendations.

OR

- **Alternative strategies:** Use strategies of an alternative equipment maintenance (AEM) program. You can do this only if the AEM program strategy doesn't reduce safety and is based on accepted standards of practice (*see* the sidebar "AEM Program" below).

AEM Program

If your alternative equipment maintenance (AEM) strategy deviates from the manufacturers' recommendations, be prepared to describe it. More to the point, be prepared to justify it: Explain how it doesn't reduce the safety of the equipment and is based on accepted standards of practice.

Elements of Your Approach

You can incorporate some critical elements into your approach to help support and justify a unique maintenance program. These include the following:

- Conducting risk assessments that involve a joint effort
- Using manufacturers' recommendations
- Referencing maintenance schedules as sources of guidance
- Reviewing maintenance history
- Seeking advice from third-party experts
- Documenting your organization's process of assessing equipment risk and frequency of maintenance

Accepted Standards of Practice

For medical equipment, accepted standards can be found in a handbook published jointly by the American National Standards Institute (ANSI) and the Association for the Advancement of Medical Instrumentation (AAMI).

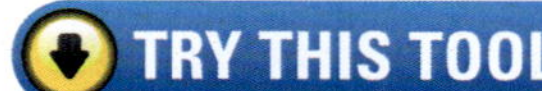

AEM Program Checklist
This checklist recommends key questions to ask when your organization assesses its alternative equipment maintenance (AEM) program's effectiveness.

Get it in writing: Whatever approach you choose to comply with, you must identify in writing (in your EC management plan) the maintenance activities and frequencies for inspecting, testing, and maintaining all medical equipment on inventory.

Manufacturers' recommendations: The manufacturers of your organization's medical equipment provide service documents with every piece of equipment. They're full of information and recommendations on maintenance, schedules, and inspections. In many cases, following them will make for a good maintenance program. But that's not always the case. Manufacturers often try to protect themselves from liability issues by recommending maintenance procedures for the most dire use circumstances. Your circumstances may be different. After the warranty expires, you may want to consider more effective maintenance approaches based on organizational risk assessments and expertise.

in other **words**

preventive maintenance (PM)

The care and servicing of equipment and utilities to help prevent failure from occurring.

Preventive maintenance strategies: Maintenance activities are essentially preventive maintenance (PM) activities. They're based on the likely failure modes of the equipment—identified in a maintenance strategy in your management plan—and on normal wear and tear. The PM types include the following:

- **Interval-based maintenance:** This popular method for PM scheduling is based on the elapsed time since the last maintenance activity. A computerized maintenance management system is typically used. This method is also known as calendar-based maintenance because it's per the calendar. The required intervals for interval-based maintenance are defined by The Joint Commission, in accord with its official time definitions (*see* "Joint Commission Official Time Definitions" on page 93).

- **Metered maintenance:** Metered maintenance tracks the actual run time or usage of a piece of equipment. A meter attached to a piece of equipment can record the hours of operation or measure the start/stop cycles. A building automation system (BAS), which can automatically track run times, stops and starts, pressure differentials, and other intervals for maintenance, would be an efficient way to adopt this method.

- **Planned-predictive maintenance:** This approach involves simple measurements (such as status/performance testing) to determine the maintenance schedule. Predictive maintenance is often used to predict the life of heating, ventilating, and air-conditioning (HVAC) equipment.
- **Corrective maintenance:** This encompasses user-requested and run-to-fail maintenance—two strategies that can be used when equipment fails and presents no risk to patients. Under user-requested maintenance, a user requests repairs to failed equipment or a replacement. Run-to-fail maintenance means running a piece of equipment until it breaks down or stops working and then simply replacing or exchanging it with a working device.
- **Reliability-centered maintenance:** This strategy involves assessing the risks associated with the equipment. You identify routine maintenance procedures and the dominant failure modes for the equipment. Then you determine the potential causes and consequences of malfunctions.

KEY CONCEPT

Medical Equipment: Responding to Failures

For Ambulatory Health Care, Critical Access Hospitals, Hospitals, Nursing Care Centers, and Office-Based Surgery

Despite the development of an effective maintenance program, medical equipment can fail. Part of your organization's program needs to include written procedures to follow when medical equipment malfunctions or fails.

Equipment replacement: Per the standards, you also need to cover how to replace equipment, including how to do that in emergency situations. Not every item of equipment requires a specific emergency response plan, but critical devices (such as ventilators) that affect the safety of patients should have planned emergency clinical interventions. This doesn't apply to laboratory settings.

Reporting equipment failure: The Safe Medical Devices Act (SMDA) of 1990 requires you to report whenever medical equipment is suspected to have caused or contributed to a person's death, serious injury, or serious illness. Health care professionals familiar with the equipment must make a judgment about the equipment's involvement, based on their user experience.

Equipment Management (EQ)

For Home Care

As you may already know, Joint Commission standards for home care accreditation apply selectively to a range of organizations that provide some or all of the following services:

- Home health—personal care and support services
- Hospice—both facility inpatient and outpatient in a patient's home
- Durable medical equipment (DME), supplies, orthotics and prosthetics, and rehabilitation technology—covering mail order items, items provided in a patient's home, and/or items provided in a facility
- Respiratory equipment and clinical respiratory services
- Rehabilitation technology
- Pharmacy

What the EQ standards cover: The Equipment Management (EQ) standards for home care required by The Joint Commission relate to medical equipment and supplies. They cover the following:
- Selection and delivery
- Setup
- Maintenance
- Backup and emergency maintenance
- Storage

Which EQ standards apply: Managing the environment of care can be challenging when the care takes place in the patient's home because the home environments vary. But some home care takes place in central facilities. Home care organizations should look at which EQ standards apply to which services and settings, using the applicability grids provided in the home care accreditation manual.

in other words

durable medical equipment (DME)

Equipment suitable for patient use outside of a medical facility and that can withstand repeated use. These items are generally not useful to an individual in the absence of a medical condition, illness, or injury. They're provided by the organization directly to the patient as sale, rental, or loaned items. Examples include, but aren't limited to, oxygen and respiratory equipment, hospital beds, bedpans, walkers, canes, and crutches.

What equipment must be managed: In most cases, your EQ management program should address the following medical equipment:
- Equipment the patient rents from your organization
- Equipment the patient purchases from your organization
- Equipment that's not provided to patients but is used only by the organization's staff

Who manages the equipment: As with medical equipment in all settings, everyone working with home care equipment needs to know this:
- How it operates
- How it's used in the care environment
- How it's maintained

Keep in mind, however, these two differences in home care:
- **Provided directly to patients:** Organizations that provide the medical equipment directly to patients manage that equipment.
- **Not provided directly to patients:** Organizations that provide medical equipment *used by the organization but not provided to patients* manage that equipment.

Selection, Delivery, and Setup of DMEPOS
Generally, organizations that supply durable medical equipment, prosthetics, orthotics, and supplies (DMEPOS) are the only ones responsible for complying with EQ standards that relate to selection, delivery, and setup.

Selecting medical equipment and supplies: Unlike many other health care organizations, home care organizations aren't required to have an interdisciplinary approach to selecting medical equipment. Still, it's always a best practice to get input from the actual users, especially when the home settings vary. The following practices *are* required:
- **Process:** You must have a process for selecting and acquiring medical equipment provided to patients.
- **Type of items:** Items you select and deliver must meet the patient's needs and limitations as well as risks involved in the patient's use of the items. You must provide only DMEPOS.

- **Regulations:** DMEPOS and other items supplied to patients must meet applicable regulations of the US Food and Drug Administration (FDA) as well as other medical effectiveness and safety standards. Also note this related requirement:
  - *Custom orthotics and prosthetics services*: You must assess the products for safety and follow the manufacturer's guidelines before fitting with or delivery to the patient. And if you have to modify or adjust them, you need access to another provider or service who can help you do that.

For Medicare patients: DME suppliers of DMEPOS to Medicare beneficiaries (patients) must provide the equipment for trial or simulation, if necessary.

Delivering and setting up medical equipment and supplies: When you're delivering and setting up items in patient homes, you need to be as accommodating as possible. You also need to keep the items (and everyone around them) safe. The standards require it. They stipulate the following:

- **Timing:** Tell the patient when delivery is expected, and make sure the time frame meets the patient's needs (as determined by the care team).
- **Transport:** Keep the items secure during transport.
- **Condition:** Make sure the items are clean, sanitary, and undamaged when they're delivered.
- **Verification:** Verify—and document—delivery of the items. This can be done for a sampling of items to a patient and might be via phone, return receipt, or copy of a delivery tracking form.
- **Risk assessment:** Evaluate whether the equipment can be used safely in the patient's home (based on electrical and environmental requirements of the equipment).
- **Assembly and storage:** You unpack it, assemble it, adjust or adapt it, perform safety and operations checks on it, and store it.

For deemed status: DME suppliers of DMEPOS to Medicare beneficiaries (patients) must meet certain additional standards related to delivery and setup, including guidelines from the American Association for Respiratory Care, and verify and document that no items are adulterated or counterfeit, were obtained by fraud or deceit, or are incorrectly branded and labeled for use. You must also make sure the time frame for setup that was agreed on is honored—even if you're working with another supplier.

Maintenance of Home Care Medical Equipment

As in other accreditation settings, the term *maintenance* encompasses inspecting and testing in addition to repairs and other maintenance activities. Unlike other settings, home care patients may be using equipment that you aren't required to maintain. Your organization needs to manage equipment it provides to the patient—by rental or purchase. But note this exception:

- Per the EQ standards, you don't have to maintain, provide backup, or provide on-call availability for equipment the patient purchases from you unless you choose to.

Summary of EQ maintenance standards content: EQ standards don't differ much from maintenance standards in other settings, but there are some distinctions. This is the gist of the similarities and differences:

- **Product information:** You need to get copies of features, warranties, and instructions from the manufacturer for every (non-custom-fabricated) item you provide to patients.
- **Maintenance guidelines:** For maintenance of equipment provided to patients as well as equipment used only by staff (for patient care, analysis, and testing), follow the manufacturer's guidelines. For safety and operation/function checks and repairs, follow the manufacturer's guidelines plus organizational policy. But note:
  - *Your own guidelines:* If the manufacturer doesn't have maintenance guidelines, your organization can establish its own. And you don't need to set up an AEM program (*see* page 95), although you can.
  - *Inspection between patients:* You have to inspect equipment between use by different patients.

- **Performance checks:** Periodically, you need to check the devices used to check your medical equipment, per manufacturer's guidelines. Other performance checks the EQ standards require involve equipment used in drug compounding and preparing.
- **Documentation:** Of course, you need to document maintenance on all equipment and performance checks.

For Medicare patients: DME suppliers of DMEPOS to Medicare beneficiaries (patients) must provide loaner equipment during repairs of any equipment owned by the patient. It must be of equal or better quality and can be provided free or for a fee.

Backup and on-call emergency equipment: In home care, it becomes pretty important to have a way to replace malfunctioning or failed equipment quickly—especially when you can't just go to another part of the building to get it. The standards cover your responsibility in detail, but here are a few summary points:

- **Life-threatening:** You need to identify equipment used by a patient that would be life-threatening if it fails or malfunctions. And then you need to provide 24/7 access to emergency services as well as backup for that equipment. For certain patients (such as those dependent on ventilators or oxygen therapy), you need to make sure the backup will last a minimum of three times as long as your organization's average response time. With oxygen concentrators, you have to consider the maximum response time, and if a patient refuses a backup oxygen concentrator, you have to educate the patient about what to do if the equipment fails.
- **Health-threatening:** You also need to identify equipment that would threaten a patient's health if it fails or malfunctions. For each item of equipment, you need to provide or arrange for backup, repair, or replacement.

Storage of Home Care Medical Equipment

Home care is exactly like other health care settings in at least one way: It involves a lot of medical equipment:

- Obsolete equipment
- Dirty equipment
- Clean equipment
- Patient-ready equipment
- Equipment needing maintenance or repair

All of this equipment needs to be (1) clearly identified and (2) stored separately at your organization's sites. Equipment—and supplies—need to be stored appropriately too, addressing things such as expiration dates, temperature requirements, and battery charge requirements.

Cleaning and cleanliness: Not only do you need separate and appropriate storage for clean and dirty equipment, you also need to clean and disinfect the dirty equipment. That should be done in a designated area. And all storage areas should be clean too—not just the areas with clean and patient-ready equipment. Finally, it should go without saying (but there's a standard that says it): You need to maintain the cleanliness of all patient-ready equipment.

KEY CONCEPT

Utility Systems: Managing the Program

For Ambulatory Health Care, Behavioral Health Care, Critical Access Hospitals, Hospitals, Laboratory, Nursing Care Centers, Office-Based Surgery, and Home Care

Utility systems are extremely important when it comes to delivering safe and reliable care to patients at your facility. When they're managed efficiently, your organization's ability to care for patients is maximized. But when problems occur, there can be severe consequences to the environment. That's why Joint Commission EC standards require you to manage risks with your utility systems, incorporating that into your EC management plan (*see* Chapter 2). But to manage those risks, you first need to know what types of utility systems are involved.

in other words

utility systems

Building systems that support the use and function of the physical environment, such as heating, cooling, water distribution, and vertical transport systems.

Types of Utility Systems

Some utility systems are common to all facilities; others may be unique to your organization. The utility systems shown below are those you may be familiar with.

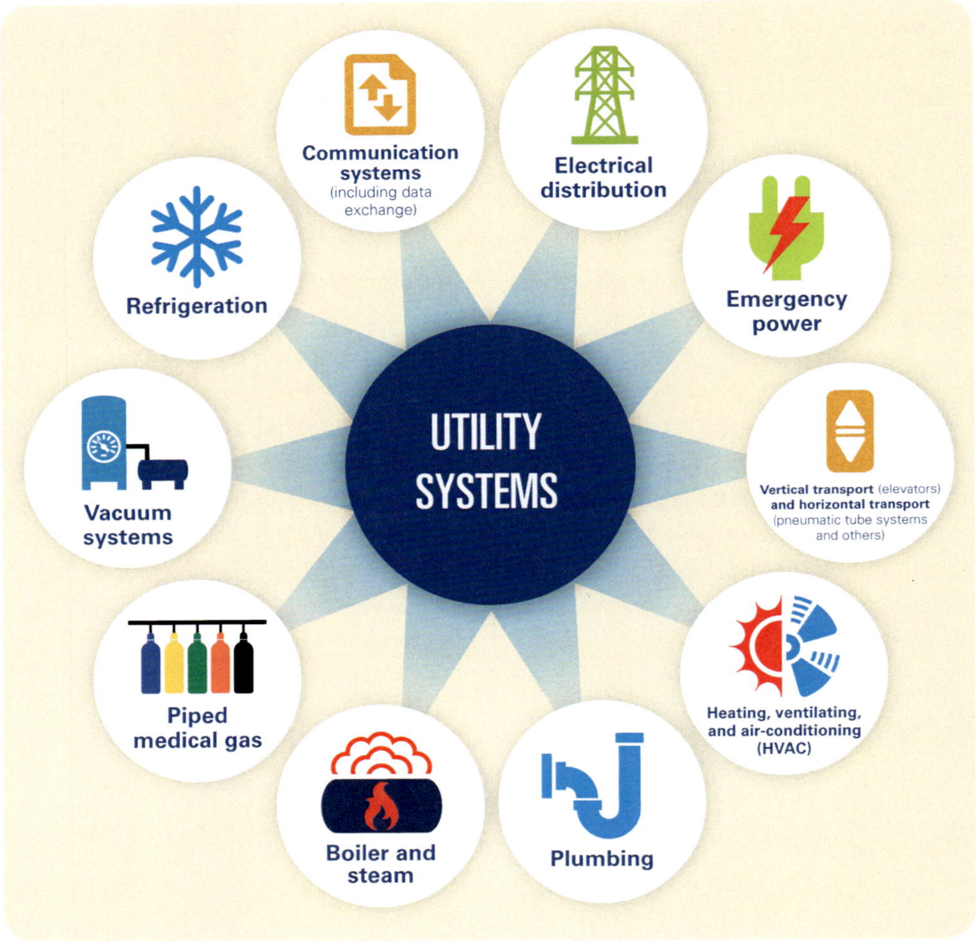

High-risk operating components: Like some types of medical equipment, certain operating components of your utility systems may be classed as *high risk* (*see* page 91). Remember, if it's high risk, it means that if the equipment or component fails, patients or staff may suffer serious injury or even death.

If they aren't your systems: If your organization is in leased or rented space, it's not directly responsible for the operation of the utilities, but it *is* responsible for making sure that the utility systems it uses are appropriate and maintained as required.

Records of utility systems inspection, testing, and maintenance should be made available to you on request.

Who manages the utilities: This can be your facilities director, office manager (for a leased space), or any other maintenance designee.

Mapping the utility systems: The Joint Commission requires you to map your utility systems (or for behavioral health care settings, have information about it). Each utility map should show where the utility system enters the building and where it runs throughout the facility. It should also show where the end points of use are and where emergency interventions can be performed, if necessary. Note that for office-based surgery, only practices that use electrical life-support equipment, provide patients with assisted mechanical ventilation, or have blood, bone, and tissue storage units are required to have utility distribution maps.

COLLABORATION: Remember that staff need to understand there's a reason behind the design of utility systems—so propping that self-closing door open, bringing in power strips from home, or not reporting utility issues or concerns can have a negative impact on the performance of the utility system. If you engage them in Q&As or discussions about their role, they'll probably respond positively. Clinical leaders, you can take the lead in modeling this, while facilities directors and accreditation professionals, you can provide guidelines and immediate feedback when any compliance violations occur related to staff use of utilities.

in other words

utility map

A drawing that shows where a utility system (such as an electrical distribution system) enters the building and how it's distributed, including end points of use, as well as emergency intervention points.

smart questions:

Who creates and updates your utility maps?

KEY CONCEPT

Utility Systems: Inventory of Operating Components

For Critical Access Hospitals, Hospitals, and Laboratory

For deemed status: *See* the sidebar "Medical Equipment and Utility Systems: Inventory and Maintenance for Deemed-Status Hospitals and Critical Access Hospitals" on page 90 for additional or different requirements related to information in this key concept.

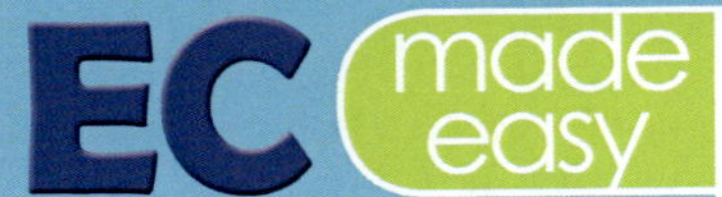

in other words

operating components of utility systems

Parts of utility systems that are performance-related and deliver a measurable outcome (such as a boiler in a heating system), but perhaps not supporting parts for those components (such as belts, pumps, and motors).

One of the best tools for managing risks is a current and complete inventory. Joint Commission EC standards require you to create a written inventory of the operating components of utility systems. As with the inventory created for your medical equipment, unless your organization is a deemed-status hospital or a critical access hospital, you have the option of using one of two approved approaches:

- **All operating components:** Inventory all operating components of utility systems.

OR

- **Selected operating components:** Inventory selected components categorized by risk.

Evaluating Risks of Utility Systems Operating Components

If you have the option to inventory only selected operating components of utility systems, you should perform a risk assessment or rank the risks. Just like you did for your medical equipment inventory (*see* page 89), rank risk criteria that include function, physical risk, incident history, maintenance requirements, and regulations and requirements.

KEY CONCEPT

Utility Systems: Maintenance

For Ambulatory Health Care, Behavioral Health Care, Critical Access Hospitals, Hospitals, Laboratory, Nursing Care Centers, Office-Based Surgery, and Home Care

For deemed status: *See* the sidebar "Medical Equipment and Utility Systems: Inventory and Maintenance for Deemed-Status Hospitals and Critical Access Hospitals" on page 90 for additional or different requirements related to information in this key concept.

Whether or not your organization owns the utilities in your facility, you have to make sure they're working properly. You can use the same maintenance strategies outlined in the section about medical equipment maintenance (*see* page 92). Any of the strategies listed (or a combination of them) will help you develop an effective maintenance program.

KEY CONCEPT

Utility Systems: Infection Control

For Ambulatory Health Care, Critical Access Hospitals, Hospitals, Laboratory, Nursing Care Centers, and Office-Based Surgery

Infections pose a serious safety risk for patients, staff, and visitors. They remain a challenge for the health care industry despite new technology, cleanliness standards, and attentive staff. When it comes to maintaining infection control, utilities can either help prevent the spread of infections or they can actually proliferate them. It's all depends on how you manage your systems. And that means monitoring and working to eliminate airborne contaminants and waterborne contaminants.

Airborne Contaminants

Biological agents (bacteria, viruses, mold), as well as gases, fumes, and construction-related dust, are considered airborne contaminants. To prevent their spread, you need ventilation equipment such as HVAC systems. The goal for HVAC in infection prevention is to provide filtration, adequate pressure relationships, and air exchange rates.

Especially sensitive areas for airborne contaminants:
Strict control of airborne contaminants is essential in areas where patients may be especially sensitive to contamination. These include the following:
- Operating rooms
- Special procedure rooms
- Delivery rooms
- Airborne infectious isolation rooms
- Protective isolation rooms
- Laboratories
- Sterile supply rooms

Maintenance of HVAC to control airborne contaminants:
A carefully designed and installed HVAC system at your facility will go a long way toward controlling airborne contaminants. But it must be maintained well to do that: It's a best practice to establish written cleaning and inspection schedules for the moving parts, including fans, coils, belts, and filters.

smart questions:

What areas of your facility have you identified as extra-sensitive to airborne contaminants?

Waterborne Pathogens

Hospitals and critical access hospitals as well as nursing care centers are required to manage waterborne pathogens such as Legionnaires' disease. These may be found in such utility components as the following:

- Cooling towers
- Air-handling units
- Potable hot/cold water systems
- Aerosolizing water systems such as showers, humidifiers, and fountains

Now, how do you identify and address the dangerous biological agents that may be hiding in your waterways?

Identifying areas most susceptible to waterborne pathogens: You may want to conduct a risk assessment to identify areas that are most susceptible to waterborne pathogens. It can also be used to determine a history of identified cases, and the status of the domestic hot water system. Check for sections of the system that have been shut off. These "dead legs" can create stagnant water where bacteria like *Legionella* (the cause of Legionnaires' disease) will most likely breed. Likewise, check areas that have been closed, abandoned, or converted to make sure water system components do not become breeding grounds for pathogens.

Addressing waterborne pathogens: Mitigation for waterborne pathogens can include installing thermostatic mixing valves to cool water down before use or delivering water to the outlets at higher temperatures. Warm water pipes between the valve and the shower should be self-draining. Cooling towers should be located in a way that allows their drift to be directed away from air intakes. Installing drift eliminators helps too, but you have to make sure to maintain them on a regular basis by keeping them clean and treated before start-up and shutdown. Water sources in abandoned spaces need to be maintained and may need to be periodically flushed (for example, closed nursing units, vacant patient rooms, or patient rooms that have been converted to offices but still have running—or stagnant—water).

COLLABORATION: Everyone knows the dangers posed by infectious disease—to patients, staff, and visitors. And everyone can help avert those dangers. Leaders, you can help spearhead or promote awareness of the need to work closely with facilities staff on this serious issue. Facilities directors and accreditation professionals, you can look for ways to make sure all facilities and clinical staff are aware of infection control protocols and how those interface with utility systems. For example, you can initiate "drill-down" interdisciplinary teams that monitor and report on dusty fan belts, pools of stagnant water, and mold on any surface.

KEY CONCEPT

Utility Systems: Piped Medical Gas

For Ambulatory Health Care, Critical Access Hospitals, Hospitals, and Nursing Care Centers

Whether it's for direct patient care or to drive medical equipment, piped medical gas and vacuum systems need your attention. Maintenance and testing of these systems and their components (area alarms, automatic pressure switches, shutoff valves, flexible connectors, outlets) should be conducted in time frames determined by the organization, according to the organization's risk assessments and the maintenance strategies outlined in this chapter. Another resource to consider is the National Fire Protection Association's (NFPA) Appendix C in NFPA 99-2012, *Standard for Health Care Facilities*.

Repairs or Breeches

When a piped medical gas system (as it's usually called) is installed, modified, repaired, or breeched in any way, you're required to test it for correct gas, gas purity, and correct pressure. According to the NFPA, staff who work on the piped medical gas system must be qualified: You don't want to risk cross-connections or contaminated gases during repairs or testing.

in other words

piped medical gas and vacuum systems
Networks of pipes that distribute medical gases or vacuum from central sources, such as tanks, throughout a facility to terminal units for access.

Labeling and Access

The Joint Commission and the NFPA expect the following for piped medical gas systems:

- **Pipe labels:** All gas piping must be correctly and clearly labeled, including what gas the piping contains.
  - *Interstitial space piping:* Piping in the interstitial space (the area between the lay-in ceiling and the roof or floor deck above), should be labeled every 20 feet with its contents.
- **Shutoff valve labels:** The main and area supply shutoff valves should be correctly and clearly labeled, including a description of the gas type located in the system and the areas the system serves.
- **Shutoff valve access:** Those working on gas systems should have unobstructed access to the shut-off valves for medical gases. This becomes especially important in an emergency situation: The valves control the flow of the piped gases such as oxygen. If there were a fire, for example, oxygen would accelerate its spread. Cutting off the gas supply quickly would be crucial to containing the blaze.

Storing medical gas cylinders: Your health care organization may provide nonflammable gases in freestanding cylinders when it's impractical to have piped nonflammable medical gases. Chapter 3 provides details on storing those safely (including correct labeling).

KEY CONCEPT

Utility Systems: Emergency Power Supply System

For Ambulatory Health Care, Critical Access Hospitals, Hospitals, Laboratory, Nursing Care Centers, Office-Based Surgery, and Home Care

Emergency power is nice to have at home, but it's necessary in all health care facilities. The Joint Commission's EC standards require health care facilities to design and install utility systems that meet their patient care and operational needs—and electricity is a big one. But what if the power goes out? That's when you need an emergency power supply system (EPSS) and/or a stored emergency power supply system (SEPSS).

---

in other words

emergency power supply system (EPSS) and **stored emergency power supply system (SEPSS)**

Systems that automatically supply emergency illumination or power to critical areas and equipment essential for safety to human life. An SEPSS has a stored energy source (battery) as part of the system. An organization may have both an EPSS and an SEPSS for a specific utility or type of equipment; in case the EPSS fails, the SEPSS is a backup system. Or an organization may have only one or the other for a specific utility or type of equipment.

Elements of an Effective EPSS

The readiness and effectiveness of your EPSS should never really be in question. You should know you're ready to go. An effective maintenance program for an EPSS covers the following:

- Essential functions that should be provided with emergency power
- Key elements of an emergency power system
- Testing procedures

Essential functions: Power is needed in an emergency for these essential functions, and the emergency power system must provide power for them within 10 seconds of an outage, per the Joint Commission standards:

- Alarm systems, as required by the *Life Safety Code®**
- Exit routes and exit signs
- Emergency communication systems
- Emergency lighting at emergency generator locations
- Elevators
- Equipment that could cause patient harm if it fails (including life-support equipment, medical air compressors, medical vacuum systems) and equipment in operating rooms, recovery rooms, and urgent care areas
- Essential refrigeration and other equipment in laboratories

Key elements: At its most basic, these are the key elements to consider in establishing an effective EPSS:

- **The power it gives:** The EPSS must provide sufficient power for essential functions in the face of any hazard. Hazards might include a generator failure, natural disaster, mass casualty event, or terrorist attack.
- **The power it gets:** The EPSS is powered by an on-site emergency standby generator of sufficient size. The fuel storage for it at your facility is based on past outages and anticipated problems caused by weather, conditions, and location.

Testing: To make sure the EPSS is functioning properly, Joint Commission standards require testing for generators and their automatic transfer switches (ATSs). Specified frequencies and durations for testing generators are stated in the standards. If the equipment fails the test, steps must immediately be taken to protect patients, staff, and visitors until necessary repairs or changes are made, and a successful retest occurs. The sidebar

* *Life Safety Code®* is a registered trademark of the National Fire Protection Association, Quincy, MA.

in other words

automatic transfer switch (ATS)

Switchgear that transfers the power from the utility to the emergency generator in the event of an electrical outage. Upon the loss of power, the transfer switch signals the generator to start. When the generator gets up to speed and produces the proper voltage and frequency, the transfer switch transfers the load to the generator.

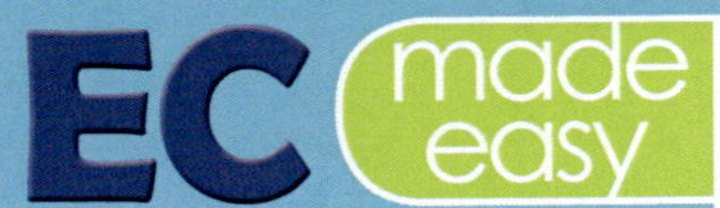

"Emergency Power Preparation" (*see* page 113) contains strategies to keep your EPSS ready to deploy.

COLLABORATION: Your organization must assume that the local community may also be compromised in a power outage, whatever the cause. If you plan to stay in operation during an outage, you need to plan accordingly, with the ability to provide utility services like electricity to the facility. Accreditation professionals and leaders, you may want to ask the facilities director for a tour of the utilities systems and the generator and talk about its testing and performance during any real or simulated emergency events. Also *see* Chapter 8 for more on emergency management.

Generator Placement and Backup

The EPSS is normally located near the spot where the electrical feed enters a building. That's usually in the lower levels of a building, such as the basement. Wherever it is, make sure the placement of generators doesn't make them vulnerable.

NFPA placement requirements: The Joint Commission currently follows the 2012 edition of the NFPA's *Life Safety Code* (*see* Chapter 7). That edition picks up a relevant standard from the 2012 edition of NFPA 99 that requires organizations to install EPSS equipment in rooms, shelters, or separate buildings that are designed and located to minimize damage.

The NFPA requirement followed by The Joint Commission is not a retroactive code, so installation locations prior to the 2012 edition standard may still be code compliant.

Backup power choices: You have to supply emergency power to essential functions (as stated previously). But you can use battery power instead of a generator to back up alarm systems, exit route illumination, emergency communication systems, and exit signage. All other items must be backed up by your emergency generator. Battery systems should provide power to supply corridor lighting for at least 1½ hours, and to alarm systems and to any equipment used in the provision of care, until normal power is restored. Storage batteries should be inspected each week and maintained according to the manufacturer's specifications.

Emergency Power Preparation

In addition to the inspection, testing, and maintenance requirements for emergency power supply systems (EPSSs), The Joint Commission supports the following proactive steps to avoid adverse events caused by an emergency electrical power system failure:

- Perform a gap analysis: Compare the critical equipment and systems needed in an extended emergency against the equipment and systems actually on the EPSS.

- Use disaster scenario planning: To better identify critical systems that could potentially be lost (for example, potable water or elevators), use disaster scenarios as you plan.

- Maintain an inventory: Document all emergency power systems and the loads they serve in a complete inventory.

- Provide training and testing: Provide training and periodic competency testing to all operators and others responsible for system maintenance of the EPSS.

- Test the generator: Run tests at least annually using American Society for Testing and Materials (ASTM) standards on the generator fuel oil, track expiration dates, and replace stale fuel oil not consumed within its storage life (or, at least annually test the fuel quality to ASTM standards).

- Let leaders know: Inform management and clinical leaders about the capabilities and limitations of the EPSS, including how long emergency power will be available, how long it will take the generators to provide power if and when the utility company's power is lost, and what locations within the facility will and won't be powered by the emergency power.

- Establish clinical contingency plans: These are for clinicians to follow during brief or sustained losses of emergency power. Include this information as part of staff orientation and periodic continuing educational activities for medical and other clinical staff.

- Be ready with battery power: Have plans in place for rapid deployment of battery-powered equipment, such as portable suction units, in case of a power failure.

- Check critical plugs: Regularly assess critical equipment to ensure that it's plugged into backup power outlets.

- Create a "disaster bin": Make one or more of these to keep on hand. Each should contain flashlights, extension cords, and so on.

Source: The Joint Commission. *Sentinel Event Alert*, Issue 37: Preventing adverse events caused by emergency electrical power system failures.

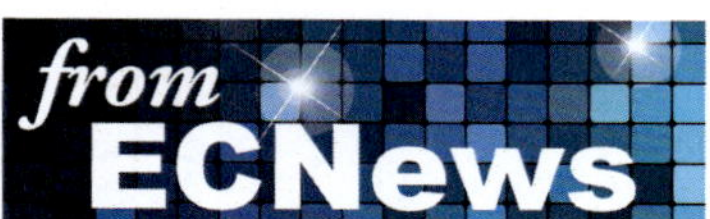

The Four-Hour Test

. . . The Joint Commission requires a four-hour run of the emergency generator every three years . . . with a load of at least 30% for diesel-fueled generators. For non-diesel-fueled generators, the four-hour test is required using the available load for the full four hours . . .

An advantage of this four-hour test is that it can assess the reliability of the entire EPSS and identify system issues. For example, one location had an emergency generator located in a basement, with a fresh air shaft alongside the generator vault. This fresh air shaft terminated 24 inches above the ground, with a large open grate to allow air movement but prevent accidental access. During a construction project, a contractor decided to place 4 x 8–foot sheets of material on the raised platform (the ventilation shaft). During the 30-minute monthly exercise, the EPSS room was not adversely affected. However, during a sustained generator run, the EPSS room, starved of make-up air with the compromised shaft, got so hot that a sprinkler head activated, causing the EPSS to fail.

—adapted from "Power Up! Keeping Emergency Power Generators On Call and Ready to Go," by George Mills, Director of the Department of Engineering at The Joint Commission, *Environment of Care® News*, January 2014

EPSS Inventory and Staff Training

Because the EPSS is so critical, it's a good idea to maintain a complete, labeled inventory of all utilities and the loads that the EPSS serves. Any operators responsible for EPSS maintenance should receive training and should be tested to make sure they can perform the steps needed to keep it running.

COLLABORATION: Accreditation professionals, you may want to check in with your facilities directors to make sure that essential functions are covered by your EPSS, working in concert with clinical leaders. Facilities directors, you need to understand the capabilities and limitations of the EPSS and communicate that to leaders before an emergency. Leaders, you need to know how long emergency power will be available, how long it'll take the generators to provide power, and what locations in the facility will and will not be powered by the emergency power. You need to communicate and collaborate now: In an emergency, it's already too late.

KEY CONCEPT

Utility Systems: Responding to Failures

For Ambulatory Health Care, Behavioral Health Care, Critical Access Hospitals, Hospitals, Laboratory, Nursing Care Centers, Office-Based Surgery, and Home Care

What if all your systems don't work? What if your backup plans don't work either? Managing utility systems not only involves assessing their reliability and maintaining them, it also means minimizing risks of their failure. Backup systems and contingency plans need to be tested frequently and regularly too. Many organizations have very old plans, created decades ago when their building was new, and haven't tested them since.

Time for a test: Plan a test at a time when the effects of a potential failure in the utility backup system are minimal so the safety of patients won't be threatened. And make sure all staff get fair warning. They'll be more ready to give feedback on the effectiveness of the test if they aren't taken by surprise. In a 24-hour care facility, you won't want to shut down everything, so you can do a mock scenario instead.

Time for a tracer: Tracers (*see* Chapter 10) can be a good way to find out who knows what about how to respond to utility failures. Whether it's part an organizationwide tracer program or an EC monitoring program, the best tracer results usually come when you tell people why you're doing the tracer and when it's planned. Sharing results of the tracers with everyone afterward helps focus them on problems the tracer highlighted. Of course, you can also do a tracer after a utility failure to find out more about how well your plans worked.

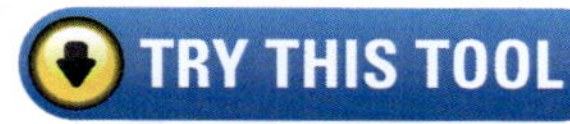

Mock Tracer Worksheet: Utility Outages
This mock tracer provides questions to ask after a utility outage in your facility.

TOOLS OF THE TRADE

- Medical Equipment and Utility Systems: Documentation Checklist
- AEM Program Checklist
- Mock Tracer Worksheet: Utility Outages

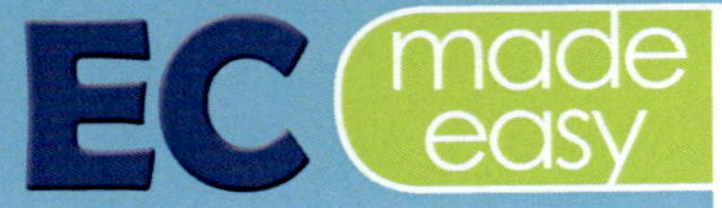

Fire Safety and Life Safety

THE BIG IDEA

A fire can be a fearsome event in any environment. But it's especially scary in a health care organization, where patients are often unable to keep themselves safe due to their illness, injury, or treatment. Also, many items in health care settings are flammable, so that threat is always looming. Fire safety and life safety are about fire protection: preventing injury to life as a result of smoke, fire, and combustion. The Joint Commission requires health care organizations to treat fire protection as a priority—from planning and practicing responses to installing and maintaining fire safety features to identifying and correcting building deficiencies.

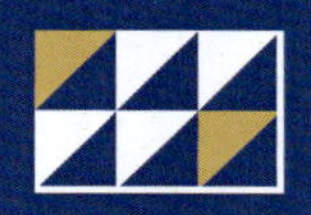

THE MANUAL

Following are the relevant Joint Commission *Comprehensive Accreditation Manual* (*CAM*) chapters:

- Environment of Care (EC)
- Human Resources (HR)
- Performance Improvement (PI)
- Leadership (LD)
- Life Safety (LS)

KEY CONCEPTS

- Fire Safety vs. Life Safety
- Fire Safety
- Life Safety
- Occupancy
- "Defend in Place" and the Unit Concept
- Statement of Conditions™

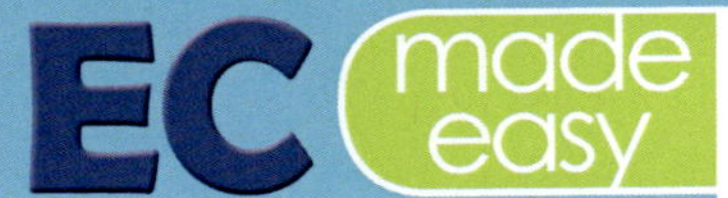

in other words

fire safety

The minimum requirements for protecting against injury to life as a result of smoke, fire, and combustion, dependent on human intervention. This includes fire drills, use of fire safety equipment, and maintenance of alarm and sprinkler systems.

life safety

The minimum requirements for protecting against injury to life as a result of smoke, fire, and combustion, dependent on building features. This includes alarm and sprinkler systems, building construction and design, maintaining means of egress, and fire protection hardware issues.

means of egress

A continuous and unobstructed way of travel from any point in a building or other structure to a public way consisting of three separate and distinct parts: the exit access, the exit, and the exit discharge.

* *Life Safety Code*® is a registered trademark of the National Fire Protection Association, Quincy, MA.

Fire Safety vs. Life Safety

In the Joint Commission standards, the terms *fire safety* and *life safety* both relate to fire protection. Standards relating to fire safety are in the "Environment of Care" (EC) and "Life Safety" (LS) chapters of the accreditation manuals; standards relating to life safety are in the LS chapters of the manuals. Both sets of standards address the minimum requirements for facility systems to offer fire protection. Note, however, that they do differ for the purposes of Joint Commission requirements, although they're interrelated.

Type of Intervention

One difference between these two sets of fire protection standards relates to the type of intervention that provides the fire protection.

- **Fire safety:** EC standards about fire safety relate to fire protection that's dependent on *human intervention*: Fire drills, use of fire safety equipment (fire extinguishers, alarm pull stations), and maintenance of alarm and sprinkler systems. They address the way people respond to and intervene in a fire situation.
- **Life safety:** LS standards relate to fire protection dependent on intervention via *building features*: Alarm and sprinkler systems, building construction and design (including location of exits), maintaining means of egress (essentially, a clear way to get out of a building from any point in the building), and fire protection hardware issues. They address how the building structure and its components work in a fire situation.

Purpose of a Facility

Another difference relates to the purpose of a facility, encompassed by the concept of *occupancy* (*see* page 131). Remember this:

- Standards in the EC chapter related to fire safety are applicable to all accreditation programs.
- LS standards are based on occupancy type because they're based on the *Life Safety Code*®.*

The Life Safety Code: As described in Chapter 1, The Joint Commission LS standards are written specifically to align with the requirements of the *Life Safety Code*, a set of national standards issued by the National Fire Protection Association (NFPA). In fact, each element of performance (EP) of the LS standards includes a reference to the *Life Safety Code*. The *Code* contains chapters for specific types of health care organizations, defined as occupancy types. Because the LS standards are also structured to reflect the structure of the *Code*, they follow the distinctions by occupancy type.

CMS and the Life Safety Code: As of November 1, 2016, both the US Centers for Medicare & Medicaid Services (CMS) and The Joint Commission began surveying to the 2012 version of the *Life Safety Code*, with the result that Joint Commission LS standards and elements of performance (EPs) will align more closely with CMS Conditions of Participation (CoPs) covering life safety.

in other words

Life Safety Code®

Requirements for building construction intended to protect occupants during fires, developed by the National Fire Protection Association (NFPA) and adopted by The Joint Commission. *Life Safety Code*® is a registered trademark of the National Fire Protection Association, Quincy, Massachusetts.

KEY CONCEPT

Fire Safety

As noted above, standards in the EC chapter related to fire safety are about human intervention for fire protection—and that doesn't just mean firefighters. All staff play a role. What those roles are should be spelled out in a written fire response plan and reinforced with training via fire drills.

Written Fire Response Plan

In addition to the requirement for a written fire safety management plan (*see* Chapter 2), Joint Commission standards require a written fire response plan. This plan describes what actions staff and licensed independent practitioners are expected to take during a fire.

Elements of the fire response plan: The plan should contain details on the following:
- **Roles and responsibilities:** Who should do what in the case of fire, covering all staff, including licensed independent practitioners, students, construction crews, and volunteers

smart questions:

What are your primary responsibilities in the event of a fire in your facility?

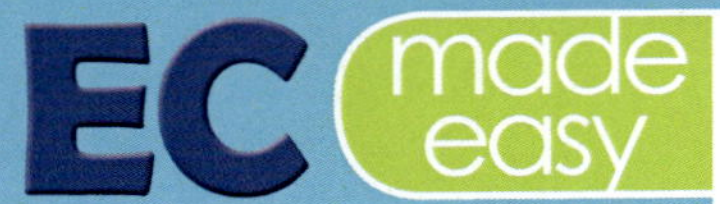

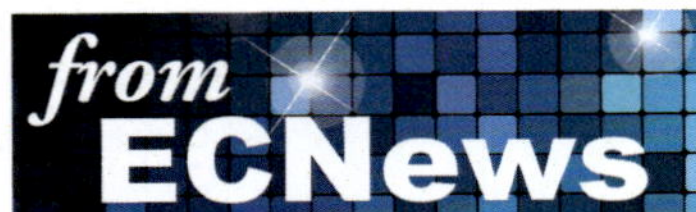

Fire Drill Training

It's critical that health care workers know what to do in a fire emergency. And they do, at least theoretically. But how many have extinguished a real fire? How many have performed a rescue from a smoky room?

Thanks to Nassau County Fire Service Academy and members of the Nassau County Fire Marshals, health care workers at St. Joseph Hospital in Bethpage, New York, have done both. During Fire Prevention Month, local fire marshals conduct training-in-action for both clinical and non-clinical staff of Nassau County's major health care facilities, including St. Joseph, a 203-bed community hospital that provides comprehensive inpatient and outpatient care. . . .

The training was developed around the RACE acronym—a series of actions for individuals who are present at a fire's source. Here's what RACE stands for:

- **Rescue**—Move anyone who is in immediate danger.
- **Alarm**—Sound the fire alarm.
- **Contain**—Close doors to contain the fire.
- **Extinguish** or **Evacuate**— If it is safe to do so, use a fire extinguisher to extinguish the fire. Otherwise, evacuate to an area behind closed smoke barrier doors.

—excerpted from "Entering the Smoky Room: Hands-On Fire Safety Training at St. Joseph Hospital," *Environment of Care® News*, March 2015

- **Responses by location:** What should be done where, including at the fire's point of origin and elsewhere in the facility
- **Special areas and populations:** What risk factors should be considered for special areas (operating room, neonatal unit) and/or for what special populations (rehabilitation patients, behavioral health patients)

Training on the fire response plan: You should know what the code is for a fire in your facility. But do you know what to do next, per your fire response plan? Staff should receive training and education on all parts of the plan, especially the sections that relate to their particular roles and responsibilities. Each individual should know his or her expected response in a fire situation and be able to carry it out if necessary.

Responding to a Fire

Your assigned roles and responsibilities for responding to a fire will usually depend on where you are when it starts or when it spreads to where you are.

Actions at the fire's source: A fire incident is particularly frightening if you're right there as it starts. It's important to take calm-but-quick action. Memory acronyms can help people remember what to do in the chaos of a real fire. Here are two commonly in use for responses at a fire's source:

- **RACE:** This is basically what you do, step by step, when you encounter a fire. It stands for the following actions:
  - *Rescue:* Move anyone who's in immediate danger, including patients and visitors—*if it's safe to do so* (the fire isn't blocking your way or spreading quickly).
  - *Alarm:* Sound the fire alarm. This will vary, and can include pulling the nearest pull station and/or calling the operator to report the situation.
  - *Contain:* Close doors (corridor doors, patient room doors) to contain the fire.
  - *Extinguish or Evacuate:* Use a fire extinguisher to extinguish the fire—again, if it's safe to do so; otherwise, evacuate to an area behind closed smoke barrier doors.

Some of these things can be done at the same time if there's more than one person present to help. For example, one person can pull the alarm while another calls the operator and others close doors.

- **PASS:** This helps you remember how to use a fire extinguisher—*if it's safe to do so*. It stands for the following actions:
  - *Pull:* Lift up the pins between the extinguisher's handles.
  - *Aim:* Point the nozzle at the base of the fire.
  - *Squeeze:* Press the handles together to spray.
  - *Sweep:* Move the extinguisher from side to side to cover the area on fire, aiming for the base of the fire.

Actions away from the fire's source: Individuals who aren't at the fire's source also have roles to play. For example, depending on your fire response plan, they should perform actions such as closing all doors to contain smoke and fire, keeping visitors with patients, preventing transport of patients, and then waiting further instruction or the all-clear announcement. (These actions are part of an approach called "defend in place." *See* page 133.)

Evacuating: If a fire can't be extinguished easily, you might need to evacuate. That can involve moving to a safer area of the building or leaving the building entirely. During an evacuation, some staff will probably be responsible for caring for patients. Others may transport patient information, like medical charts. Of course, these roles should be predetermined in your fire response plan, and staff should receive relevant training. (*See* above sections and Chapter 8 for more on evacuation.)

Shutting off medical gas: Another action that may be required is shutting off medical gas, such as a patients' oxygen supply. This might, however, put patients at risk. So it should be done only in particular situations, such as when a fire is spreading or there's an explosion. Because it can be a complex task, the responsibility is usually assigned to someone who has—or should have—special training (knowing when it's appropriate

smart questions:

Who has the authority and training to shut off medical gases per your fire response plan?

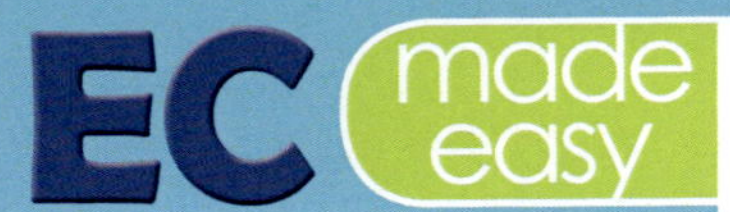

and providing portable backup tanks). That person(s) may be different, depending on the location in your organization and your occupancy type. Surveyors will ask, "Who has the authority and training to shut off medical gases, per your policy?" You need to know the answer to that question. Placing a sign at or near the medical gas valve can help staff remember what the protocol is and who is authorized to turn off the medical gas zone valve.

Fire Drills

Fire drills are an indispensable activity. They are used both to practice responding to a fire and to identify which parts of the fire response plan could use improvement.

When to conduct fire drills: According to Joint Commission standards, an organization defined as a health care occupancy (*see* page 131) should conduct a fire drill at least once per shift every quarter. Other occupancies have similar requirements; see your applicable accreditation manual for specifics. Don't forget days and times should be varied.

Who should be involved in fire drills: All staff should be actively involved in fire drills and know their roles. The standards specify the number of drills required and when to perform them. A common goal in organizations is to make sure that all staff are able to participate in drills. In order to include more staff in the drills, you can conduct evening and night drills via a coded announcement to avoid disturbing patients but make sure all the elements of your drill are completed (for example, signal has been sent to central station monitoring company). Also, with the adoption of the 2012 *Life Safety Code*, in lieu of an audible alarm signal, visible alarm appliances can be used. Don't forget weekend and fire drills in special areas such as the operating room (usually during annual training), the kitchen (according to the NFPA, the number one location for fires in health care), the loading dock, the MRI suite, and so on.

Unannounced fire drills: Starting in January 2018, *all* of your organization's fire drills should be unannounced. Unannounced drills give the most accurate picture of what's probably going to happen in a real fire situation. They also prevent preplanning of staff responses. In some areas, such as an operating room or intensive care unit, though, it's better to give staff a few minutes' notice of a drill. This allows individuals involved in sensitive work to continue without disruption.

Evaluating fire drills: The fire drills should be evaluated in a predetermined, structured way. Here's what evaluation should entail:

- **Staff:**
  - After each drill, evaluate staff response during the drill.
  - After each drill, provide additional training and education, if necessary.
  - Annually, evaluate staff knowledge of what to do in a fire situation, whether or not staff participated in a drill during the previous year.
- **Equipment:** After each drill, evaluate performance of fire safety equipment during the drill.
- **Evaluation methods:**
  - *During the drill:* Observers strategically located throughout the facility can record their observations.
  - *For annual evaluations of staff knowledge about fire response:* Quizzes or role play can be used.
- **Documentation:** Document all parts of the evaluations.

COLLABORATION: Accreditation professionals, note that fire drills are one area of the environment of care in which you may take a lead, such as helping to train the staff on the fire response plan. Facilities directors, you'll work with the accreditation professionals and department-level leaders—as well as community firefighters—to schedule, conduct, and evaluate the drills. Leaders—and this includes EC staff and clinical staff leaders—you need to understand your role in fire response, which may involve participation in the drills or performing the evaluations.

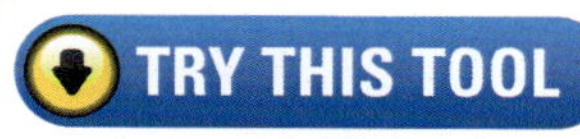

Sample Fire Drill Matrix
You can use a form like this to help track your organization's fire drills and ensure variation between shifts and days.

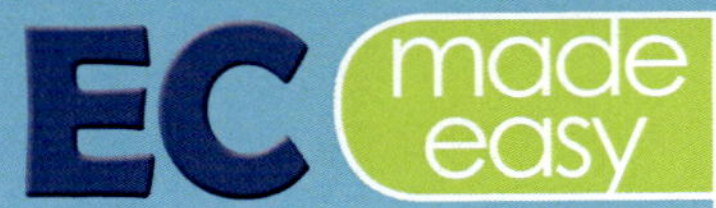

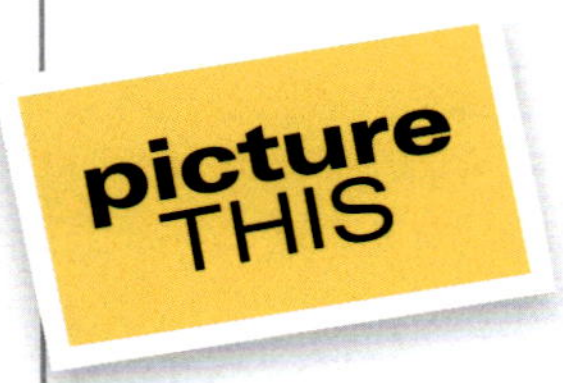

Sample Completed Fire Drill Matrix

Day = M, Tu, W, Th, F, Sa, Su

COMPLETED FIRE DRILL Matrix

Shift			Q1			Q2			Q3			Q4		
			Jan.	Feb.	Mar.	Apr.	May	Jun.	Jul.	Aug.	Sep.	Oct.	Nov.	Dec.
Shift 1st	Normal	Location		4TH						8TH			11TH	
		Day		THUR.						THUR			TUES	
		Date		2-26-15						8-27-15			11-24-15	
		Time		0800						08.45			0830	
	ILSM	Location					5TH							
		Day					5-28-15							
		Date					Thurs.							
		Time					0854							
Shift 2nd	Normal	Location			3RD			6TH			9TH			BASEMENT
		Day			Thur			Thur			Thur			TUES
		Date			3-25-15			6-25			9-24-15			12-29-15
		Time			1650			1700			1630			1710
	ILSM	Location												
		Day												
		Date												
		Time												
Shift 3rd	Normal	Location	1ST			2nd						10TH		
		Day	Friday			Tues						Friday		
		Date	1-30-15			4-28-15						10-30-15		
		Time	0540			0520						0600		
	ILSM	Location							7TH FL					
		Day							Tues					
		Date							7-28-15					
		Time							0530					
Weekend	Normal	Location												
		Day												
		Date												
		Time												
	ILSM	Location												
		Day												
		Date												
		Time												
Other MRI OR ?	Normal	Location												
		Day												
		Date												
		Time												
	ILSM	Location												
		Day												
		Date												
		Time												

A fire drill matrix can pull together information from several sources and in so doing help you see patterns. Collecting all the days, dates, and times in one place makes it very clear when there is a lack of variation. As you can see, three of this hospital's four first-shift fire drills were conducted on Thursday mornings, and all four were between 8:00 A.M. and 9:00 A.M. Similarly, the second-shift fire drills were almost all on Thursdays at about the same hour of the day. This hospital did not vary its fire drill schedule very well, and would be considered in noncompliance.

Fire Safety Equipment Inspection, Testing, and Maintenance

Whether your organization is big or small, you probably have at least some of the following fire equipment and fire safety building features:

- Visual/audible fire alarm devices
- Sprinklers
- Dampers
- Smoke/heat detectors
- Pull stations
- Fire extinguishers
- Standpipe systems
- Fire/smoke barrier doors

If you're big, you probably have A LOT of these! Note that The Joint Commission doesn't require you to have it all. But for those items you do have, Standard EC.02.03.05 tells you which ones you need to inspect, test, and maintain, and how often.

Schedules: Each type of equipment has different requirements for inspection, testing, and maintenance. Visual and audible fire alarms, for example, must be tested every 12 months. The accreditation manuals include notes that point to NFPA sources on how to perform tests. Managing all the testing and maintenance on schedule can be overwhelming, but you just have to do it to maintain a safe environment—and document that you did it.

Documentation: All EPs for this standard—and there are many—require documentation. For some pieces of equipment, such as portable fire extinguishers, the documentation can be done using a bar code system, check marks on a tag, or an inventory (*see* Chapter 6).

COLLABORATION: Facilities directors, when you're reviewing the documentation for inspection, testing, and maintenance, make note of how each EP is scored. Accreditation professionals, you'll want to look at this documentation at a high level and talk with facilities directors about solving any chronic noncompliance issues.

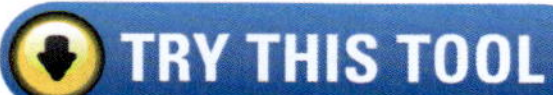

Fire Safety Equipment and Building Features Documentation Checklist
You can use a form like this to check your documentation of your fire safety equipment and building features inspection, testing, and maintenance.

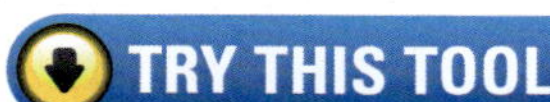

Checklist for Compliance with Standard EC.02.03.05
This checklist can help your organization determine compliance with EC.02.03.05 and target areas for improvement.

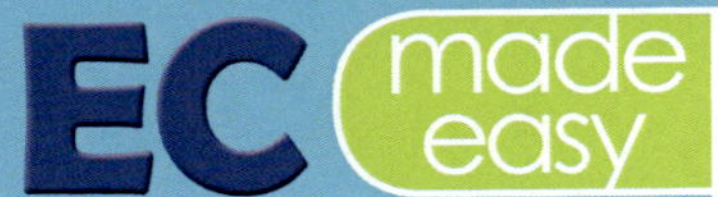

in other words

building assessment
Established process to assess compliance with the *Life Safety Code* and self-identity deficiencies in the building environment. Building assessments also establish corrective action measures. Time frames may be established by the organization; however, annual is recommended.

barrier
A separation made up of walls, doors, windows, and so on, intended to prevent the spread of fire or smoke.

fire rating
A classification indicating a material's resistance to fire, usually stated in terms of the time it takes for fire to burn through the material.

Life Safety

As explained earlier in this chapter, the *Life Safety Code* and related Joint Commission LS standards address the building features used for fire protection. Organizations are required to evaluate compliance with building features during regular building assessments. The primary building features addressed are barriers, corridors, and doors. Following are some basic issues to be aware of for each feature.

Barriers

Barriers are separations typically consisting of walls and the features within walls (doors, windows), but not all walls are barriers. When it comes to the *Life Safety Code*, there are two kinds of barriers:

- **Smoke barriers:** These contain smoke and restrict its movement.
- **Fire barriers:** These protect occupants from fire itself and the products of combustion.

Fire rating: Fire barriers have a fire rating based on the length of time they're effective in fire containment. Fire *protection* ratings are applied to doors and windows; fire *resistance* ratings are applied to walls (*see* the sidebar "Fire Ratings" on page 128).

Protection: In smoke or fire barriers, any openings—doors, windows, above-ceiling conduits, cables, pipes—must have protection to prevent passage of smoke and/or fire, depending on the barrier being reviewed (existing vs. new, smoke vs. fire). To be effective, barriers must have protection from outside wall to outside wall, and from floor to ceiling or roof. Access to these barriers should be limited to avoid inadvertent breaches, which include holes (also known as "penetrations"). In the case of any breach—accidental or purposeful, the barrier must be properly repaired using proper materials to maintain protection. Smoke compartments provide areas of refuge for horizontal movement and must be identified on drawings. Note that smoke compartment requirements vary for new and existing occupancies.

Doors

In a health care facility, a door isn't just a door. What it is and what it's called depends on its purpose—such as preventing the spread of fire or smoke. Most doors are also necessary for maintaining egress—a primary directive of the *Life Safety Code*.

Doors in barriers: Doors are obviously necessary, but they pose life safety concerns because when they exist in smoke and fire barriers, they create a breach. In the *Life Safety Code*, each opening must be protected by an opening protective. Doors are an opening protective. (Openings in elevator shafts or laundry chutes are among the other types of openings that need opening protectives.) Here is the minimum you need to know about doors in barriers:

- **Fire barrier doors:** Like all fire barriers, these doors are fire-rated. They must also have self-closures or automatic-closing devices, and those are required to latch. Do not remove any hardware because this will invalidate the door rating, and make sure labels are legible! Don't forget that doors on your linen and trash chutes require a fire rating.
- **Smoke barrier doors:** These must have self-closures or automatic-closing devices but ARE NOT required to latch— IF the wall in question is just a smoke barrier. If the wall serves more than one purpose—smoke and fire barrier, it DOES have to latch.

Propping doors open or disabling latching mechanisms negates the barrier's effectiveness. Regular, thorough inspection and maintenance, including the required annual inspection and testing, can help ensure that doors are working the way they're supposed to. Your life safety drawings (*see* page 137) will provide guidance on what doors you have, so you can check them against the requirements.

in other
words

opening protective
A device such as a door used to protect an opening in a wall used as a fire or smoke barrier.

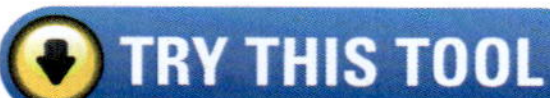

Quick-Look Door Check
You can use this tool to perform compliance checks on fire and smoke barrier doors as well as corridor doors.

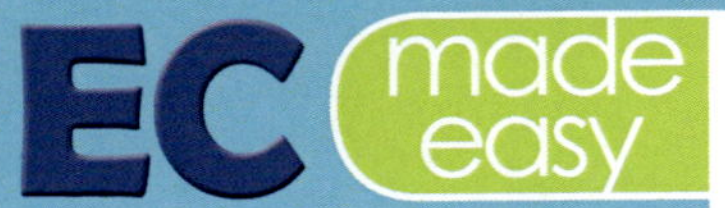

Corridor Clutter: Clearing the Means of Egress

The means of egress must be free of clutter. The three components of the means of egress (the exit access, exit, and exit discharge) must be free of impediments to the public way. This includes equipment and materials in the corridor and snow/ice on the sidewalks outside. However, exceptions exist:

Carts and equipment in use (not in storage). Items considered to be in storage could include items in the egress corridor that have not been used for more than 30 minutes.

Other exceptions are allowed when the organization provides at least 5 feet of clear and unobstructed corridor width, including the following:

- Crash carts, because these are always considered to be "in use"
- Wheeled equipment, including chemotherapy carts and isolation carts (while associated with patient care delivery)
- Transport equipment, including wheelchairs and gurneys
- Patient lift equipment, including, for example, when the organization has patient lift outside of every room

Exceptions also exist for fixed furnishings, provided that the compartment is fully protected with smoke detection or is in direct supervision of staff. Also, the furnishings must not reduce

(continued on page 129)

Fire Ratings

These terms are used when discussing fire ratings in the Life Safety standards and the *Life Safety Code*®:

- **Fire door assembly:** A fire barrier that consists of any combination of a fire door, a frame, hardware, and other accessories that together provide a specific degree of fire protection to an opening.
- **Smoke door assembly:** A smoke barrier that consists of any combination of a door, a frame, hardware, and any other accessories that together restrict smoke movement through door openings by limiting the amount of air that can pass through the assembly.
- **Fire protection rating:** The designation that indicates the duration of the fire test exposure for a fire door assembly or fire window assembly in which it successfully met all NFPA criteria (per NFPA 252, *Standard Methods of Fire Tests of Door Assemblies*, or NFPA 257, *Standard on Fire Test for Window and Glass Block Assemblies*). Normally used to describe a fire door assembly.
- **Fire resistance rating:** The time, in minutes or hours, that materials or assemblies have withstood a fire exposure (as determined by the tests, or methods based on tests, prescribed by the *Life Safety Code*). Normally used to describe a fire wall or fire barrier wall.

Rating or No Rating?

- Not all walls are required to have a fire resistance rating, and not all doors are required to have a fire protection rating. Whether a wall requires a rating, and consequently whether any openings in that wall require a rating, depends on a combination of factors, including the following:
  - Occupancy type (*see* page 131)
  - Hazard level (per purpose and size of the room)
  - Whether the building is protected with automatic sprinklers

Source: *NFPA Glossary of Terms*, June 2012, National Fire Protection Association, Quincy, MA.

Locked doors and maintaining egress: One of the main objectives of the *Life Safety Code* is to make sure there are clear and unobstructed means of egress. That usually means keeping doors unlocked. However, in some cases, you need locked doors for clinical or security reasons. This is true in areas housing psychiatric, obstetrics, and Alzheimer's and dementia patients. There are very specific regulations in the *Life Safety Code* that outline exactly which doors may be locked and in what fashion. These guidelines may help:

- **Locking procedures:** Locking procedures may include delayed-egress locking mechanisms, key-operated locks, or a combination.
- **Quick unlocking:** In all cases, staff must be able to quickly unlock any locked doors whether with a key or badge. (Delayed egress and access control doors have special requirements, so check your accreditation manual.)
- **Staff and keys:** In the case of key-operated locks, the key must be carried by the staff person—not kept at the nurses' station or in a lock box. Fire safety plans must identify which staff members will have keys.
- **Common keys:** Also, all doors should be keyed the same or be operable by key cards or badges to avoid delays caused by fumbling for the right key.

Corridors

Medical equipment, mobile computer workstations, and food service carts: These items are common culprits in the dangerous habit of corridor clutter. Corridors are how people move from one place to another. In the event of a fire situation, people have to be able to move quickly and easily away from the fire. Obviously, that's not possible if corridors are cluttered. Wheeled equipment (such as equipment and carts currently in use, equipment used for patient lift and transport, and medical emergency equipment not in use) is allowed if at least five feet of clear and unobstructed corridor width is maintained, provided there is a fire plan and training program addressing its relocation in a fire or similar emergency.

30-minute rule: Certain items, such as emergency medical equipment (for example, crash carts, isolation carts), in-use equipment (such as equipment required by patients), and patient lift and transport equipment (if certain conditions are met) are allowed in corridors. No other items may be stored (left unused for 30 minutes) in corridors—including patients.

Air flow and fire: Corridors also present concerns about air flow. Where air goes, so go smoke and fire. To help keep smoke and fire out of corridors, ventilation systems that use corridors for air supply, air return, or air heating and cooling aren't allowed.

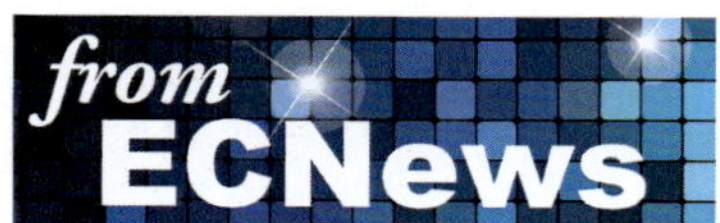

(continued from page 128)

the corridor width below 6 feet, must be on one side of the corridor, and must not exceed 50 square feet. Groupings of fixed furnishing must be kept at least 10 feet apart. At no time can fixed furnishings restrict access to fire protection or building service features. The furnishings must be securely attached to the wall or floor. For example, if a nursing unit had stroke patients that needed exercise and were encouraged to walk the corridor with a walker, fixed seating could offer respite for the patient.

—adapted from
"Understanding Key Changes to the Life Safety Standards"
by George Mills, Director of the Department of Engineering at The Joint Commission
Environment of Care® News,
June 2017

Exceptions to the Rule

Among the new requirements and exceptions stipulated in the US Centers for Medicare & Medicaid Services (CMS) final rule are the following:

- Roller latches on hazardous area and corridor doors are banned.
- An ambulatory surgery center is regarded as ambulatory health care if one or more of its patients is incapable of self-preservation.
- A fire watch or evacuation of the facility or affected portions of the building must transpire if the fire alarm system is out of service for 10 out of 24 hours or a sprinkler system is out of service more than 10 hours in a 24-hour period in an occupied building.
- CMS may waive particular provisions of the *Life Safety Code®* due to circumstances of unreasonable hardship.
- Every sleeping room must contain an exterior window or door for buildings constructed 60 days following adoption (after approximately September 9, 2016); the height of the fixed window sill cannot exceed 36 inches above the floor (some exceptions apply).
- Alcohol-based hand rub (ABHR) dispensers may be installed by hospitals, so long as the installation adequately safeguards against inappropriate access. In addition, the projection of the dispenser may not exceed 6 inches.
- All buildings taller than 75 feet (high-rises) must be equipped with required automatic sprinkler protection by 2028.
- Organizations must abide by the 2012 *Life Safety Code*'s new chapter (no. 43) on building rehabilitation.
- Chapters 7, 8, 12, and 13 (on information technology, plumbing, emergency management, and security, respectively) of NFPA 99-2012 have been extracted.

KEY CONCEPT

Occupancy

"What's your occupancy type?" That's really the first question you need answered in any discussion of the *Life Safety Code*. The answer to that determines which parts of the *Code* apply to your organization. The *Life Safety Code* has different requirements for compliance based on a facility's purpose, known as its occupancy.

Incapable of self-preservation: The explanations of occupancies that follow make reference to individuals who are "incapable of self-preservation." What does that mean? In terms of the *Life Safety Code*, it means being unable to get up and walk out of a burning building due to any of the following: age, physical or mental disability (including conditions related to medical treatment, such as with an obstetrics patient), or because of security measures not under their control. A key determination in occupancies is the *number* of persons who are incapable of self-preservation *simultaneously* (at any one time).

Relevant Occupancies

Four types of occupancies are relevant for Joint Commission purposes:

- **Ambulatory care**
  - ***Purpose:*** Provides services or treatment to four or more patients* at the same time that requires (1) treatment that renders them incapable of self-preservation; or (2) anesthesia that renders them incapable of self-preservation; or (3) emergency or urgent care that, due to the nature of their illness or injury, renders them incapable of self-preservation. Note that in this occupancy type, the individuals' incapacity must be caused by the treatment or care being provided.
  - ***Length of stay:*** Less than 24 hours
  - ***Examples:*** Ambulatory surgery centers seeking accreditation for Medicare certification (*see* the manual for clarification of ambulatory program classification) and freestanding ambulatory, emergency, or urgent care centers.

---

in other words

occupancy

In life safety, the purpose for which a building or portion of a building is used or meant to be used. Depending on the organization, occupancies may include ambulatory health care occupancy, business occupancy, health care occupancy, and residential occupancy

---

* For CMS deemed ambulatory surgical centers, the definition applies when one or more patient is provided services.

- **Health care**
  - *Purpose:* Provides medical or other treatment or care of persons suffering from physical or mental illness, disease, or infirmity; and for the care of infants, convalescents, or infirm-aged persons.
  - *Length of stay:* 24 hours (overnight) or more
  - *Examples:* Inpatient facilities such as hospitals, critical access hospitals, nursing homes, and limited care facilities
- **Residential**
  - *Purpose:* Provides sleeping accommodations for normal residential purposes for individuals capable of self-preservation and includes all buildings designed to provide sleeping accommodations. They're known in the *Life Safety Code* as lodging and rooming house occupancy (16 or fewer occupants) and hotel and dormitory occupancy (17 or more occupants).
  - *Length of stay:* 24 hours (overnight) or more
  - *Examples:* Inpatient residential treatment facilities, which are generally accredited as behavioral health care organizations
- **Business**
  - *Purpose:* Provides outpatient care, treatment, day treatment, or other services where there are three or fewer people whose treatment renders them incapable of self-preservation
  - *Length of stay:* Less than 24 hours
  - *Examples:* Freestanding office-based surgery practices or laboratories

Application of LS standards: The LS standards apply to any organization classified as a health care, ambulatory, or residential occupancy. Freestanding business occupancies aren't surveyed to the "Life Safety" (LS) chapter of the accreditation manual. However, business occupancies must still comply with EC standards related to fire safety.

smart questions:

What are the occupancy types of each of the facilities in your organization?

KEY CONCEPT

"Defend in Place" and the Unit Concept

The many concepts within life safety are nuanced and complex, but they all have a clear purpose: helping you to save lives in the event of a fire. Understanding these next two is critical to fulfill that purpose.

Defend in Place

Whereas business occupancies may evacuate during a fire, allhealth care occupancies are expected to "defend in place." This means that patients who are incapable of self-preservation (*see* page 131) can depend on the staff and the building itself to protect them *where they are* while emergency personnel respond to the situation. Staff responsibilities in an actual fire were outlined above, as were the various life safety components necessary to defend in place: barriers, doors, and corridors. The building's structure and how those components are arranged within it play equally important roles.

The Unit Concept

In the world of fire protection, you can think of structures as arranged according to a unit concept. This is not a term used in the *Life Safety Code*, although it is related to *compartmentation*, which is. In the unit concept system, the facility is divided into nested units of defense. The goal is to contain the fire and smoke in as small a unit as possible. The details will vary by the type of occupancy.

Units of defense in health care occupancies: For health care occupancies, there are five general units (or levels) of defense, as follows (and pictured on page 135 in "Units of Defense: Health Care Occupancies"):

- **Unit 1 — Room:** The smallest unit of defense in a health care facility is a room. In a sprinklered environment, due to the rapid response of the sprinkler, the patient room is also the first unit of defense. The most effective defense at room

in other words

defend in place

An emergency fire strategy for health care occupancy in which occupants remain within the health care facility rather than be evacuated. This is accomplished by limiting the development and spread of a fire emergency to the room of fire origin and reducing the need for occupant evacuation, except from the room of fire origin.

unit concept

A method of constructing a facility that aims to contain fire and smoke through compartmentation features (consecutive units of defense) and provide a safe means of egress.

in other words

compartmentation

Using building components (barriers, doors, corridors) to allow staff and patients to "defend in place" in the event of a fire, both to prevent the spread of fire and to provide a safe means of egress.

smoke compartment

A space within a building enclosed by smoke barriers on all sides, including the top and bottom.

horizontal evacuation

Moving individuals to an area of refuge beyond closed smoke or fire barrier doors—as opposed to *vertical evacuation*, which involves moving individuals to a lower floor or out of the building.

level is the area being "sprinklered." Because individual patient rooms are not required to be separated from each other by fire and smoke barriers (per the *Life Safety Code*), nonsprinklered rooms don't provide much protection or containment, but the wall that separates the room from the corridor does, so it has to be fire-rated in a nonsprinklered building.

- **Unit 2 — Compartment:** Using barriers, doors, and corridors to create compartments that can contain fire and/or smoke is known as compartmentation, or smoke compartmentation (a compartment unit is based on the size of a smoke compartment). It's one of the most important features in the *Life Safety Code* because it allows staff to do a horizontal evacuation to an adjacent compartment that's protected. Horizontal evacuation is often enough to ensure safety and can prevent the need for you to evacuate your entire facility.

- **Unit 3 — Floor assembly:** Floor assemblies vertically separate occupancies into floors. A floor assembly unit contains a fire-rated floor slab and all vertical penetrations of that slab. Floor assemblies create barriers that prevent fire and smoke from spreading vertically. Any vertical openings (elevator shafts, stairways, laundry chutes) should be protected with "opening protectives" (*see* page 127)—and that includes any access panels required for wiring and such. Here's one reason why floor assembly units are so important: If horizontal evacuation fails on any one floor, vertical evacuation is the next option.

- **Unit 4 — Building structure:** The entire building structure—columns, girders, trusses, bearing walls—is the largest unit of defense. It must be able to withstand the effects of a fire long enough to allow staff members to defend in place. Key elements in that goal are the exterior load-bearing walls and floor and roof construction. The height of the building determines, by regulation, how long it has to maintain its structural integrity in a fire.

Units of Defense: Health Care Occupancies

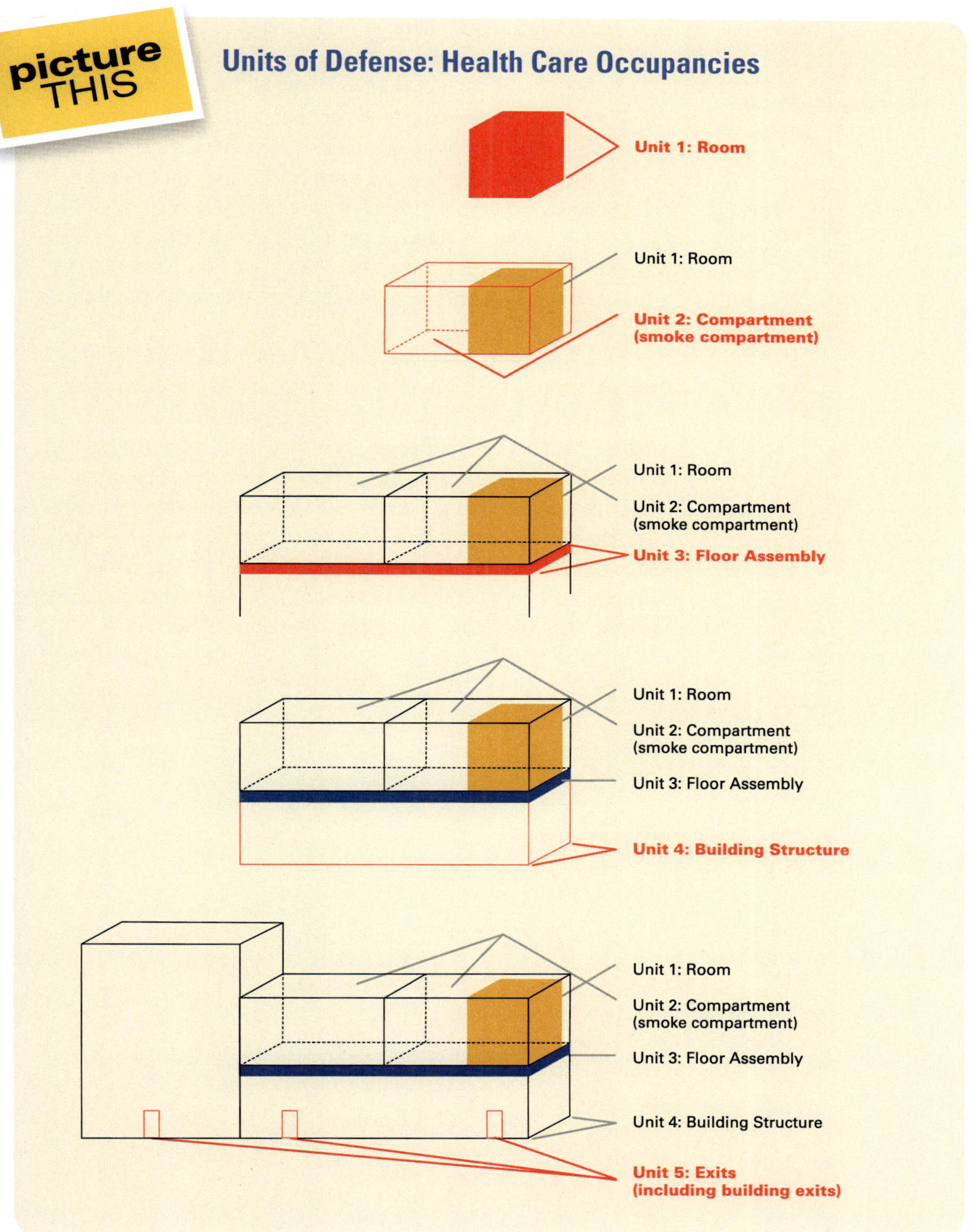

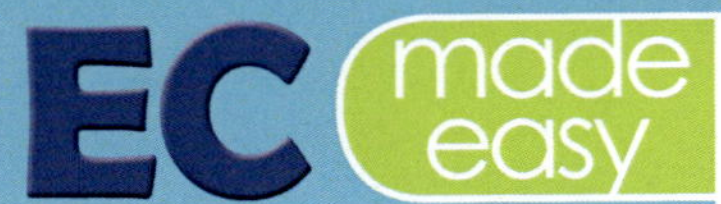

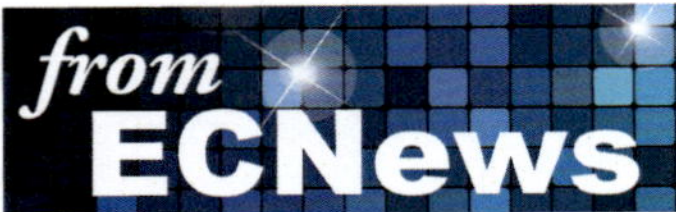

Protecting Storage Areas from Fire

Certain areas of a health care facility present more risks for fire than others. For example, storage areas can contain large amounts of material that can burn during a fire, such as supplies, equipment, and laundry. To protect occupants of a building from fire hazards associated with high-risk areas, these areas have certain fire protection requirements. For example, in storage areas of nonsprinklered existing buildings [in health care occupancies], perimeter walls must extend from the floor to the deck, be of one-hour fire-rated construction, and include a 45-minute fire-rated door that latches and closes automatically. In sprinklered storage areas of existing buildings [in health care occupancies], perimeter walls must resist the passage of smoke and have doors that latch and close automatically. For new construction [in health care occupancies], storage rooms larger than 100 square feet must have perimeter walls that are one-hour rated and doors that self-close and latch.

—excerpted from "Understanding Fire and Smoke Protection Features: Examining the 'Life Safety' (LS) Chapter," by George Mills, Director of the Department of Engineering at The Joint Commission, *Environment of Care® News,* March 2010

- **Unit 5 — Exits:** Properly functioning exits are the final unit of defense. Exits enable people to move between compartments within the building, and outside the building if necessary. In a "defend-in-place" occupancy like a health care occupancy, building evacuation is rare, but it's still possible. The basic requirement for each floor is at least two approved exits from the space, located remotely from each other. When someone enters an exit area and leaves an unsafe environment, that person is considered safe. Clearly, exit areas are a priority in a preventive maintenance program.

COLLABORATION: Staff and clinical leaders, you should know the areas of refuge in your organization. In most cases, if a fire occurs, you'll be helping coordinate a horizontal evacuation of patients in your immediate area to an adjacent compartment. However, extreme cases may require the entire population of a building to evacuate to a location outside the facility. Accreditation professionals and facilities directors, you need to make sure leaders—and everyone else—understand the related concepts of "defend in place" and the unit concept, and make sure that's part of your fire response plans.

KEY CONCEPT

Statement of Conditions™

To help organizations meet the requirements of the *Life Safety Code* and related LS accreditation standards, The Joint Commission developed an electronic tool known as the Statement of Conditions™ (SOC), available on your *Joint Commission Connect*™ extranet site (*see* Chapter 10). If your organization is a health care occupancy, you need to maintain a current SOC. It has the following sections:

- **Basic Building Information (BBI):** This is an optional demographic review of building occupancies and related information, as identified in your organization's Electronic Application for Accreditation (E-App). Although no longer mandatory, an updated BBI can be used to describe fire safety features, like sprinklers and alarm systems.

- **Plan for Improvement (PFI):** Basically, this is a now-optional plan for correcting any self-identified EC and LS deficiencies and maintaining continuous compliance. Each PFI outlines specific activities planned to fix the problem, a target date for completion, and tracking of progress. It's meant to be a living document, updated until the deficiency is fixed.

- **Survey-Related Plans for Improvement (SPFIs):** This is a plan to correct and maintain any surveyor-identified EC and LS deficiencies. Organizations must respond to the SPFIs in the SOC to identify the corrective actions that must and will be taken within 60 days to show Evidence of Standards Compliance (ESC). (Chapter 10 has more on SPFIs.)

Life Safety Drawings

The optional BBI is where you should indicate where you keep current life safety drawings that identify the locations of life safety features. Current LS drawings must include the following:

- **Legend:** A legend that clearly identifies all features of life safety (pictured on page 139 in "Detail of a Life Safety Drawing")

- **Sprinklered areas:** Areas of the building that are fully sprinklered (if the building is partially sprinklered)

in other words

Plan for Improvement (PFI)

A optional plan to manage and correct an organization's self-identified deficiencies of the *Life Safety Code*® (*see* Chapter 10).

Survey-Related Plan for Improvement (SPFI)

A plan to address an organization's noncompliance with aspects of the *Life Safety Code*®, as identified in the Life Safety Assessment portion of the on-site survey (*see* Chapter 10).

Evidence of Standards Compliance (ESC)

A report that a surveyed organization must submit within 60 days after a survey in which it receives a Requirement for Improvement (RFI) for an accreditation requirement. The report must detail actions taken to bring the organization into compliance with each requirement, or explain why the organization believes it's in compliance. The report has to address compliance at the element of performance (EP) level.

life safety drawings

Accurate and current maps included in an organization's Statement of Conditions™ (SOC) that show sprinklered areas of the organization's buildings, barrier locations, suite boundaries, and other fire and life safety features, as well as approved equivalencies and waivers, as per Joint Commission requirements.

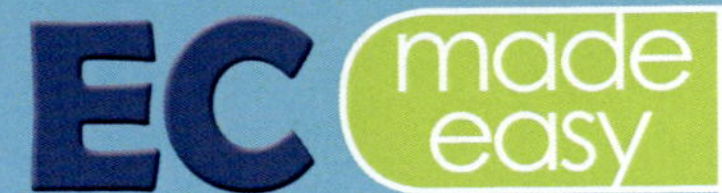

**in other
words**

interim life safety
measures (ILSMs)

A series of 11 administrative actions designed to temporarily compensate for significant hazards caused by an organization's construction activities, or when there are deficiencies related to the *Life Safety Code*®.*

* *Life Safety Code*® is a registered trademark of the National Fire Protection Association, Quincy, MA.

- **Locations of hazardous storage areas**
- **Locations of barriers:** All rated barriers, smoke barriers, and designated smoke compartments
- **Suite boundaries:** Indications of the size of the identified suites—both sleeping and nonsleeping
- **Locations of chutes and shafts:** Elevator, laundry, and other vertical openings
- **Any approved equivalencies or waivers**

Interim Life Safety Measures (ILSMs)

When you create a PFI or SPFI, you have to determine whether special temporary measures are needed to ensure safety until the situation is resolved. These are known as interim life safety measures (ILSMs). There are 11 ILSMs. Because the ILSMs most frequently come into play during construction, they are further listed and described in Chapter 9. Currently, if The Joint Commission surveyor finds an instance of noncompliance with the Life Safety standards, the organization must implement an ILSM until the deficiency is remedied, unless it can resolve the issue while surveyors are still on site.

ILSM assessment: Not all deficiencies require ILSMs. But you have to assess every compliance issue to determine if it *does* require any. If it does, the details about which ILSMs you need go into the PFI or SPFI. For example, suppose that a portable x-ray machine bangs into a door. The door is dented so it won't close completely. The organization's PFI or SPFI describes the situation and explains that a replacement door has been ordered. It also states that the new door will take two months to arrive. The ILSM assessment determines that this particular situation doesn't require any additional measures to maintain safety until the new door is installed because the door is neither a fire-rated nor a smoke barrier. When the project is completed, the PFI or SPFI is updated to reflect the resolved situation.

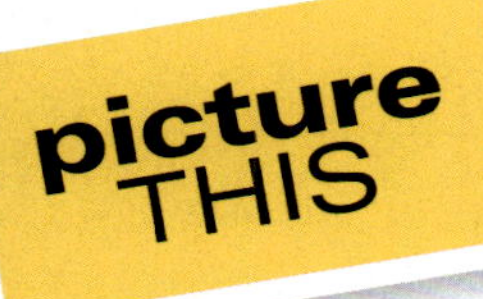

Detail of a Life Safety Drawing

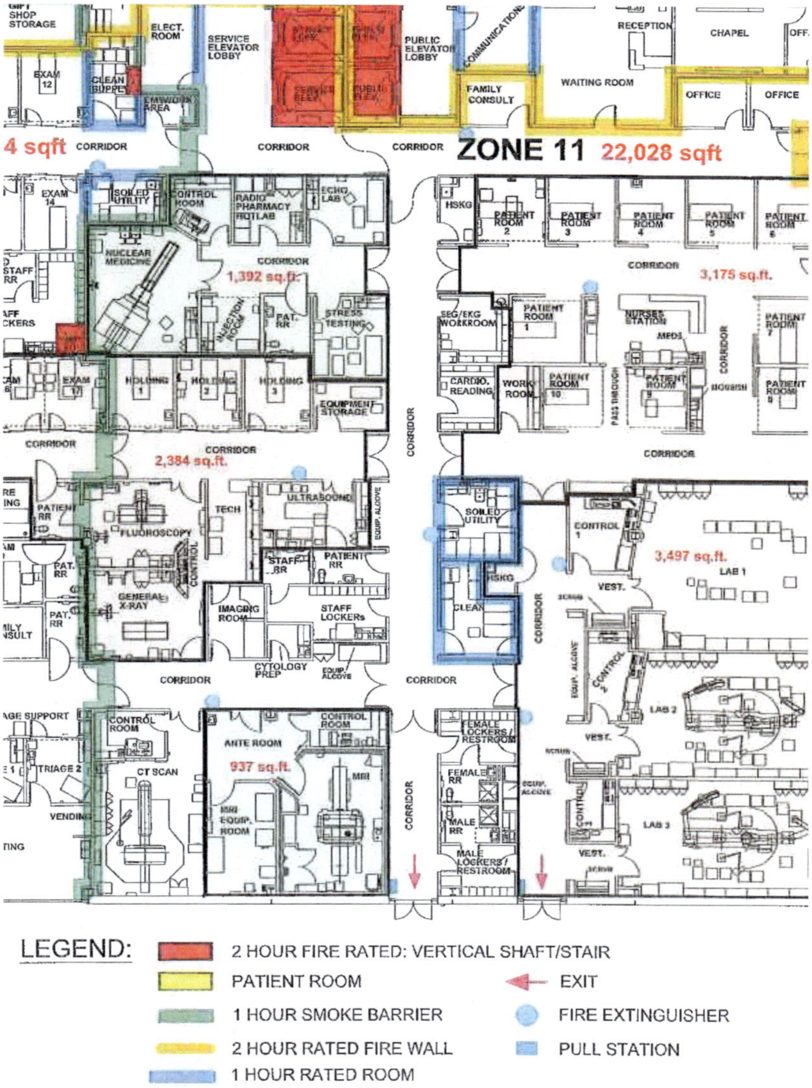

LEGEND:

- 2 HOUR FIRE RATED: VERTICAL SHAFT/STAIR
- PATIENT ROOM
- 1 HOUR SMOKE BARRIER
- 2 HOUR RATED FIRE WALL
- 1 HOUR RATED ROOM
- EXIT
- FIRE EXTINGUISHER
- PULL STATION

LS.01.01.01, EP 3, requires organizations to maintain accurate life safety drawings, like this one. As you review them with your facilities staff, check that they contain all of the Joint Commission requirements, including locations of smoke compartments.

Copyright AMITA Health Adventist Medical Center Hinsdale, Hinsdale, IL. Used with permission.

in other words

equivalency

A Joint Commission–approved alternate approach to a known *Life Safety Code* deficiency that is mitigated by other building features so that the noncompliant condition is no longer identified as deficient. The Joint Commission has two types of equivalencies, a Traditional Equivalency and a Fire Safety Evaluation System (FSES) equivalency. The Traditional Equivalency requires field validation by a registered architect, a fire safety professional, or a fire marshal responsible for community fire safety. The FSES is a formula-based approach that evaluates the entire building and deducts deficient conditions. If the net score is 0 or better, the building is considered "equalized." Both types of equivalencies require submittal to and review by The Joint Commission. When The Joint Commission completes its analysis, the request is forwarded to the appropriate Centers for Medicare & Medicaid Services (CMS) regional office for final disposition.

Equivalencies

You have several other options for addressing *Life Safety Code* deficiencies that can't be fixed immediately, including use of an equivalency (a Joint Commission–approved alternate approach) or a time-limited waiver (*see* Chapter 10). Equivalencies are used when major construction or other difficult-to-meet conditions would be necessary to correct a deficiency.

For deemed status: CMS has to approve all life safety equivalencies for hospitals and critical access hospitals.

TOOLS OF THE TRADE

- Sample Fire Drill Matrix
- Fire Safety Equipment and Building Features Documentation Checklist
- Checklist for Compliance with Standard EC.02.03.05
- Quick-Look Door Check

Chapter 8

Emergency Management

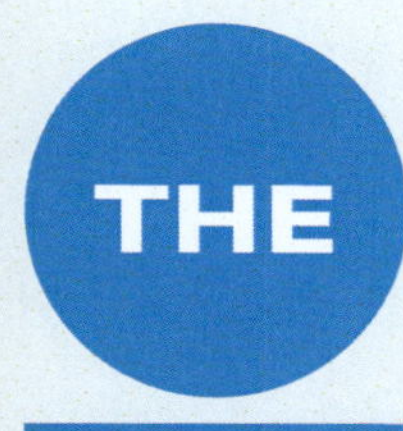
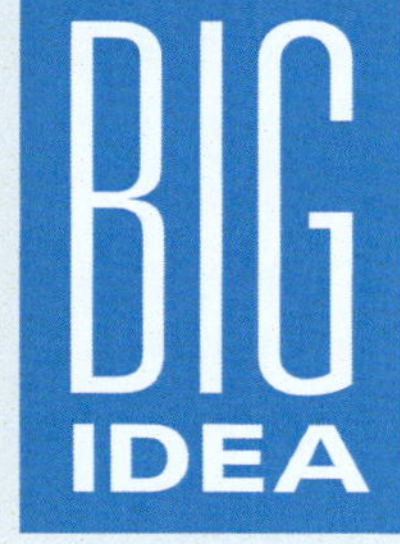

Whether it's a hurricane, an influenza outbreak, or a terrorist attack, emergencies can cause widespread human suffering and tax a community's resources. Your health care organization must adequately plan for managing these emergencies to protect your patients and staff as well as the communities you serve. Emergency management (EM) involves myriad moving parts, including performing a hazards risk assessment, creating and maintaining an Emergency Operations Plan (EOP), prepping for different phases of emergency response, training staff, establishing an incident command system (ICS), coordinating efforts with the community, and practicing emergency exercises.

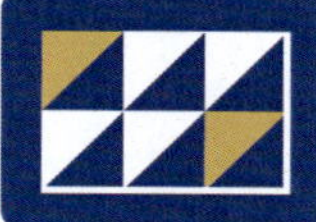

THE MANUAL

Following are the relevant Joint Commission *Comprehensive Accreditation Manual* (*CAM*) chapters:

- Emergency Management (EM)
- Leadership (LD)

KEY CONCEPTS

- Leadership Accountability in Emergency Management
- Hazard Vulnerability Analysis
- The Four Phases of Emergency Management
- The Emergency Operations Plan
- The Six Critical Areas of Response
- Incident Command System
- Community Networking
- Emergency Response Exercises
- Evacuation
- Cyber Emergencies

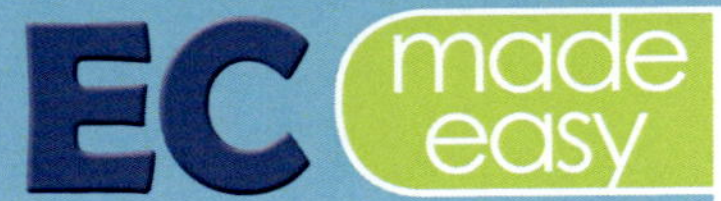

KEY CONCEPT

Leadership Accountability in Emergency Management

Leaders set expectations, develop plans, and implement procedures. That skill set is vital when it comes to preparing for and responding to an emergency. Emergency management not only requires expert planning but also commitment to implementation with sufficient resources.

Appointing an Emergency Risk Manager

One of the things high-level leaders do is appoint someone to manage risks in the environment of care (*see* Chapter 1). That person is usually the safety officer. But for emergency management, your leaders may appoint others to this role instead, such as an emergency manager and/or a quality manager. In any case, the safety officer and whoever is appointed to manage risk as part of the emergency management process should work together to pool knowledge about emergency-related risks and hazards that may arise in the environment of care. Although organization leaders must drive and remain engaged in the emergency management planning process, Joint Commission standards do not require the CEO, administrator, or other leaders to actually coordinate the ongoing emergency management processes after they have been established.

Leading an Emergency Management Team

Emergency management requires teamwork. Whoever is appointed the emergency management leader should also be the leader of an interdisciplinary emergency management planning team. For this, you need to bring in key people from within and outside the organization—representatives from all the organization's facilities and departments, as well as the safety officer. The team leaders can direct the formation of emergency response teams too, each with an appointed leader. Other health care organizations in your system, community or coalition, public health, public works and public safety partners, and other community agencies can all play an important role in supporting the organization's preparedness and resilience.

COLLABORATION: Leaders, as part of setting expectations for emergency management, you need to foster and promote staff participation—a crucial element. Facilities directors, safety officers, and accreditation professionals, you'll have to make sure facilities and clinical staff are ready to be involved. That means helping to organize training, emergency response exercises (*see* page 158), and other activities that require organizationwide cooperation.

LD Requirements for Emergency Management

In the hospital and critical access hospital accreditation program settings, the Joint Commission Leadership (LD) standards address leadership accountability for organizationwide emergency management. Leaders are required to identify an individual to be accountable for the following:

- Staff implementation of the four phases of emergency management (*see* page 146)
- Emergency management across the six critical areas of response (*see* page 150)
- Collaboration among clinical and operational areas to implement emergency management organizationwide (critical access hospitals only)
- Identification of and collaboration with community response partners
- Establishment of priorities for performance improvement in emergency management

Participating in planning: Leaders, including leaders of the medical staff, are also expected to participate in planning activities. These should take place prior to developing an Emergency Operations Plan (EOP) (*see* page 149).

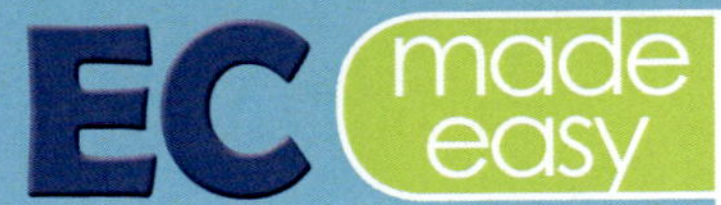

KEY CONCEPT

Hazard Vulnerability Analysis

Have you done an HVA? The first order of business for emergency management is to conduct a hazard vulnerability analysis (HVA). It identifies the potential emergencies your organization is most likely to face in your community or region. And it identifies the impact of those on your organization's ability to provide care, treatment, and services to your patients. Make sure you review the HVA with local EM leaders and officials.

HVA Requirements

Joint Commission Emergency Management (EM) standards focus on preparation for "hazards, threats, and adverse events." These are essenitally emergencies that might also include disasters. The EM standards require you to do the following:

- Conduct an HVA.
  - Identify emergencies that could affect demand for services.
  - Identify the likelihood of those emergencies occurring.
  - Identify consequences of those emergencies.
- Prioritize the emergencies in the HVA in collaboration with the community.
- Use HVA findings to define preparedness activities.
- Share with local EM officials.

Consider a range of events: Planning for every possible emergency may not be feasible or realistic, but try to evaluate as many threats as possible—both natural and man-made. These include internal events like a power outage, fire, or cyber attack, and external events such as ice storms, pandemics, or commuter train crash. Some emergencies involve an influx of patients (industrial accident requiring mass decontamination), other emergencies result in damage or destruction to the organization's physical environment (tornado).

Tailored to your area: You should tailor your HVA to your geographic area, looking at realistic natural and human threats. Are you vulnerable to hurricanes? Forest fires? Blizzards? Are you situated near a chemical factory that might be the source of a major accident? Or near a major freeway, convention center, or stadium that might be a terrorist target?

Developing and Maintaining an Effective HVA

An effective hazard vulnerability analysis (HVA) doesn't just happen. Here are some suggested steps to help you develop one:

➤ **Step 1 — Gather the team:** Host a brainstorming session with organization experts and representatives.

➤ **Step 2 — Generate a list:** List potential emergencies. Make sure they're realistic for your region.

➤ **Step 3 — Review historical data:** Look at information on emergencies over the past few decades in your region. Move to the top of the list any emergencies that have occurred previously in the community and/or the health care organization.

➤ **Step 4 — Determine probability of occurrence:** For each type of emergency, determine the probability of occurrence. Make adjustments to the list order based on likelihood of occurrence.

➤ **Step 5 — Assess impact:** Assess how each emergency would affect the organization and reorder accordingly.
  – If lives could be lost and safety is threatened, the emergency should move up on the list.

  – Evaluate the long-term effects of each emergency as well. For example, an influx of contaminated patients might require taking the emergency department offline for a long period of time.
  – Consider also how the organization's reputation could be damaged by a lack of preparedness.

➤ **Step 6 — Conduct a gap analysis:** To determine likely emergencies that you aren't prepared for and the steps to fix that, conduct a gap analysis.

➤ **Step 7 — Do a community review:** Review the HVA with other emergency response agencies and health care organizations in the community to identify common risks and threats.

➤ **Step 8 — Participate in community preparedness:** To test your strategies, participate in community planning and emergency training activities.

➤ **Step 9 — Review annually:** Review the HVA annually as a team.

How to Conduct an HVA

You can conduct an HVA in many ways. Some organizations, for example, use a quantitative scoring method to rank potential emergencies. The key is for you to identify, list, and rank the hazards you most likely need to be prepared for. You might consider following the steps described in the sidebar "Developing and Maintaining an Effective HVA" above.

smart questions:

When was your last HVA conducted? Who was involved? What was the process used?

COLLABORATION: A multidisciplinary team is best for creating your HVA. Why? Different members of the team will have varying viewpoints on the possible impact and level of preparedness associated with different risks. For example, accreditation professionals, you may be on the team due to compliance concerns. You might think that an electrical power outage would be a catastrophic issue for the facility. However, facilities directors or safety officers, you could clarify that it wouldn't be that bad, because of the backup power systems; however, a water outage could shut down the entire institution in a short period of time. Working together, you can shape the organization's response efforts.

The Four Phases of Emergency Management

For every emergency prioritized in the HVA, you must consider the four essential phases of emergency management activities: mitigation, preparedness, response, and recovery. These four phases occur over time.

EMERGENCY

Mitigation Preparedness   Response   Recovery

Phase 1 — Mitigation

Mitigation includes any activities that can be performed to minimize the probability, severity, and/or impact of an emergency *before* it actually occurs. Mitigation starts with identifying hazards and then assessing the vulnerability of patients and staff, the facility and key organizational functions, to those hazards. Mitigation activities are designed to strengthen, harden, and reinforce organizational capabilities so that they can withstand the impact of emergencies, maintain essential patient care functions, and provide a safe environment for patients and staff.

Phase 2 — Preparedness

Preparedness relates to activities that will organize and mobilize essential resources for effective emergency response. Preparedness goes beyond planning, it requires the organization to take active steps in advance to provide for the key capabilities that are essential for delivering patient care safely in an emergency. Regardless of the type of emergency, the key areas are as follows:

in other words

mitigation

Actions taken in attempting to reduce the probability, severity, and/or impact of a potential emergency; first of the four phases of emergency management.

preparedness

Actions taken to build capacity and identify resources that may be used if an emergency occurs; second of the four phases of emergency management.

- Communications
- Resources and assets
- Safety and security
- Staff
- Utilities
- Patient clinical and support services

Preparedness actions include the following:

- **Resources inventory:** Creating an inventory of resources that might be needed in an emergency, including prearranged agreements with vendors and health care networks to fulfill that inventory
- **Staff training:** Staff training on general emergency response procedures, for those with specific roles in emergency response
- **Exercises:** Conducting organizationwide exercises to test the plan (*see* page 158)
- **Ongoing planning:** Maintaining an ongoing planning process that incorporates lessons learned and process improvements identified in exercises and responses to actual emergencies

Phase 3 — Response

The response phase is put into effect during an actual emergency or during an exercise. In this phase, the organization activates its EOP (*see* page 149) and the response procedures developed in the preparedness phase, including activating the incident command center (*see* page 154). Response addresses primary and secondary impacts.

Primary impacts: Most fundamentally, response involves providing care, treatment, and services to victims, employing triage, as necessary, to address the primary, initial impacts of the emergency. Depending on the scope of the organization's services and capabilities, response procedures can include a range of responses, including the following:

- Maintaining or expanding services
- Conserving resources
- Curtailing services
- Supplementing resources from outside the local community
- Closing the organization to new patients
- Conducting staged or total evacuation (*see* page 161)

in other words

response

Actions taken when an emergency occurs; third of the four phases of emergency management.

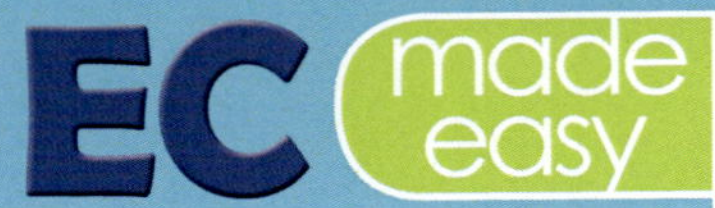

Secondary impacts: Emergencies can be complex, or evolve over time, so anticipating secondary impacts to the organization is an important aspect of situational awareness. A secondary impact is one that may not be prevalent in the initial effects of the emergency. For example, loss of a utility may have immediate effects on the organization, such as loss of power. The secondary impact is that air-conditioning isn't connected to emergency power because it can drain the system. If it's hot outside, that increasing heat level in the facility can now impact services, such as canceled surgeries, patient health in which increased temperatures can have a negative impact, and overheating equipment.

Phase 4 — Recovery

The recovery phase involves restoring the organization to normal operations and resuming the usual care, treatment, and services. Recovery may also result in returning operations to a "new" normal. A variety of important factors need to be considered for recovery. These include the following:

- **Finances:** What are the financial implications of the emergency? Can you continue to support all current services as well as planned initiatives for the near future?
- **Services:** What affect has the emergency had on your scope and range of services? Do you need to contract with outside services for help?
- **Staffing:** Do you have all the staff you need to keep delivering safe, high-quality care, treatment, and services? Were any staff injured during the emergency? Are routes to the facility blocked? Do you need to readjust staff schedules?
- **Staff concerns:** What are the concerns of affected staff? Do they need child care, elder care, pet care, mental health care, or special needs care?
- **Insurance:** Do you have coverage for what just happened? Do you have the documentation you need to file claims in a timely way?
- **Inventory:** Do you have sufficient supplies to get through an emergency (*see* page 151)? Do you have ways to get more supplies if some are damaged? Do you have supplies to repair damages?

in other words

recovery

Actions taken to restore services after an emergency; last of the four phases of emergency management.

- **Repair:** What structures or equipment need repair or replacement? Can you repair damaged items on site?
- **Authorization:** Do you have management authorizations for purchasing, document security, and outsourcing of services that temporarily cannot be provided internally?

Recovery time and complexity: The length and complexity of this phase depends on whether the emergency is ongoing as well as whether the facility itself is affected and the local area or region is still affected. How well and how quickly you recover can also be impacted by how quickly the event occurred— a hurricane with advance warning or a plane crash with no warning.

KEY CONCEPT

The Emergency Operations Plan

The HVA is an important risk management document. It's also the jumping off point for the creation of another critical document: The Emergency Operations Plan (EOP).* The EOP is a written document that an organization creates to help structure its efforts for the four phases of emergency management. It serves as a blueprint for managing care and safety during a crisis.

What an EOP Should Do

In brief, for most organizations, your EOP should do the following regarding emergency response activities:

- **Describe the ICS:** Explain in detail the organization's chain of command and decision-making authority for emergencies. This includes triggers for initiating incident command and opening the incident command center, and notifications to staff and leadership that incident command has been initiated (*see* page 154).
- **Identify roles and responsibilities:** Identify who will be responsible for what in the clinical, operational, administrative, and support areas throughout the organization.
- **Describe response procedures:** Describe in detail the response procedures that will be executed and the required staff, supplies, and space that will be activated in response

in other
words
Emergency Operations Plan (EOP)
An organization's written document that describes the process it would implement for managing emergencies that could disrupt the organization's ability to provide care, treatment, and services. (Called an Emergency Management Plan in behavioral health care.)

* Behavioral health care organizations create an Emergency Management Plan (EMP) instead of an EOP, but they're similar in intent. The organization's structure and the functioning-level of the populations it serves will determine the complexity of its EMP.

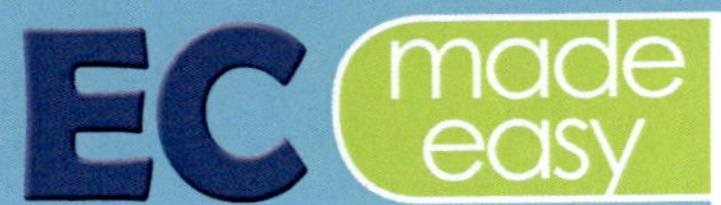

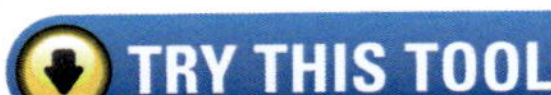

Sample Emergency Operations Plan Contents
You can compare your own EOP against this sample EOP contents to assess whether you're capturing everything you need to in your plan.

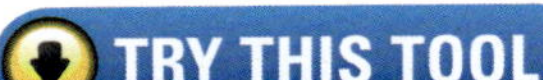

96-Hour Operational Impact Chart
This spreadsheet will help you keep track of supplies during 96 hours of emergency operation.

to the emergency. Detail how each of the key capabilities will be utilized in emergency response: Communications, resources and assets, safety and security, utilities, staff, patient clinical and support activities. Identify specific community and/or other health care organizations that will participate in your emergency response activities.

- **Determine alternative care sites:** If your organization isn't able to provide care, treatment, and services, the emergency plan should document the alternative care sites with which you have established relationships and agreements for patient care during emergencies.
- **Identify resources:** Per Joint Commission standards, if your organization plans to remain open, you need to assess your capabilities and resources to determine whether you can be sustainable for 96 hours without reliance on community resources.

96-hour requirement: Note that organizations with the 96-hour requirement are *not required to stockpile supplies to last for 96 hours of operation.* Also, although the EOP doesn't require organizations to conduct emergency exercises that actually last 96 hours, you should conduct exercises that rehearse and plan strategies for when you cannot be supported by the local community for an extended time (*see* page 157).

The Six Critical Areas of Response

Regardless of the cause or type of emergency, there are essential capabilities in a health care organization that must be protected in order to provide safe patient care and sustain essential facility functions. Because of this, the EM standards for ambulatory health care, behavioral health, critical access hospital, hospital, laboratories, nursing care centers, office-based surgery, and home care programs focus on performance in critical functions of response in the EOP. Check your accreditation manual to see which of these six functions are required in your setting.

Communications

The organization needs to identify in the EOP how it will communicate during an emergency (using phones, two-way radios, HAM radios, social media and online tools, and other means) with the following:

- Employees and licensed independent practitioners
- Authorities in the community (police, fire department, health department)
- Patients
- Media
- Suppliers
- Other health care organizations and alternative care sites

Resources and Assets

Personal protective equipment (PPE), water, fuel, staff, medical supplies, and pharmaceuticals are all resources and assets vital to emergency response. Consequently, your EOP should explain how you'll do the following during an emergency:

- Acquire supplies, PPE, medications, and more
- Interface with suppliers to create emergency supply plans
- Collaborate with outside organizations to share supplies
- Identify local, regional, and federal stockpiles
- Monitor consumption of internal supplies throughout emergency response and recovery

Safety and Security

You need to maintain a protected and safe environment for patients and workers during an emergency. Start by explaining in your EOP how you'll do the following:

- Specify internal and external security arrangements
- Control the movement of people in and around the facility
- Manage the flow of vehicles trying to access the facility
- Define the roles of external security agencies (police, National Guard, FBI)
- Effectively contain and dispose of hazardous materials and waste
- Isolate and decontaminate patients exposed to biological, chemical, and radioactive contaminants (*see* the sidebar "Isolation and Decontamination" on page 152)

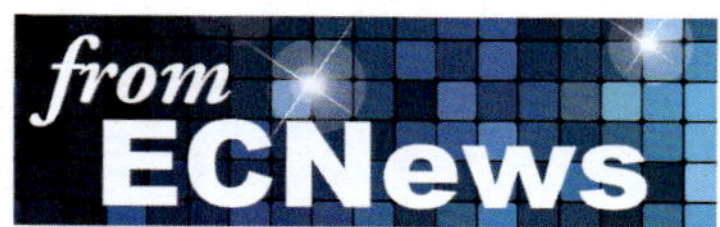

Thinking Ahead About Disaster Volunteers

When disaster strikes, hospitals and health systems sometimes need to ramp up their staffing rapidly. Patient census increases, extended shifts, potential personnel shortfalls, and other evolving dynamics all combine to create a demand for help—in a hurry. Depending on the situation, organizations may choose to bring volunteer physicians, nurses, and other clinicians into the facility when the Emergency Operations Plan (EOP) has been activated and the organization is unable to meet immediate patient needs. The organization choosing to use clinical volunteers during an emergency must identify in advance who will be responsible for assigning disaster privileges or responsibilities to the volunteers. During the actual emergency, the organization will vet their credentials, and delineate their responsibilities to make sure they're qualified to provide care throughout the emergency; forward-thinking organizations have implemented processes where they proactively credential practitioners so that when a disaster hits, they can quickly bring in volunteers to provide care and help the hospital navigate the emergency.

—adapted from "Effectively Mobilizing Emergency Volunteers: Distinguishing Between Disaster Privileging and Assigning Disaster Responsibilities," *Environment of Care® News*, December 2014

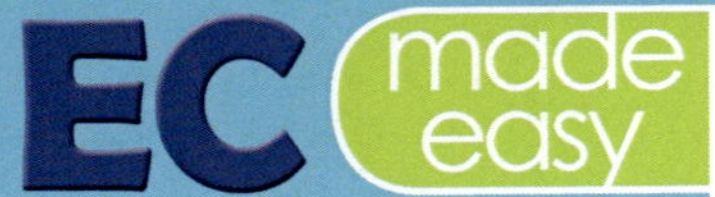

Staff Responsibilities

So much depends on staff during an emergency. In your EOP, address staff responsibilities by doing the following:

- Identifying and defining staff and volunteer roles
- Devising a clear reporting structure
- Providing effective staff training
- Providing for support for staff and their family members (housing, food and water, transportation, stress debriefings, mental and religious support, child/elder/pet care)
- Implementing a method for identifying staff and authorized volunteers (cards, badges, wristbands)

Isolation and Decontamination

In a catastrophic event involving biological, chemical, or radioactive substances, health care organizations must be ready to act quickly in isolating and/or decontaminating people exposed/affected. Basic approaches to each are provided below.

Isolation

- Provide a barrier between workers and patients by having employees don personal protective equipment (PPE)
- Segregate patients from staff, including preparing patient rooms for airborne isolation, negative pressure, and separation of air intake and exhaust.

Decontamination

- Be prepared with a well-trained hazardous materials and waste (hazmat) response team that's ready with supplies of portable units to decontaminate those affected. You can't just rely on community hazmat teams.
- Establish a decontamination area either outside or within the main facility (provided there's a direct entrance from the outside and a separate ventilation system that exhausts directly to the exterior of the building) to prevent further contamination.

Utilities Management

Your organization needs to address the possibility that one or more utilities (fuel, water, medical gas and vacuum systems, electricity, wireless technology, battery backup systems, vertical/horizontal transport systems) will be unavailable during an emergency. Plan in your EOP for alternate means of providing these utilities.

Patient Clinical and Support Activities

Most importantly, your EOP must address how to manage patients during an emergency. Address factors such as the following:

- Patient scheduling, triage, assessment, treatment, admission, transfer, and discharge
- Documenting and tracking patients' clinical information
- Personal hygiene and sanitation needs
- Vulnerable populations (geriatric, pediatric, special needs individuals)
- Mental and spiritual health needs
- Mortuary services
- Horizontal and vertical evacuation of patients (if necessary)

A common and comprehensive approach: Focusing on the critical areas in your EOP can help you better prepare for emergencies and take an "all hazards" approach to emergency management: The EOP response procedures address the prioritized emergencies but are also adaptable to other emergencies that your organization may experience. In addition, this common and comprehensive approach supports planning across organization types in systems and in health care coalitions. All settings—hospitals, ambulatory health care, home health, behavioral health, nursing care centers, and laboratories—must focus on the critical areas. In so doing, they can collaborate across settings and build mutual support and resilience through joint planning, training, and exercises on a common platform. Examples of collaboration across settings include the following:

- Hospitals receiving patient transfers from nursing homes in wildfire impacted areas
- Ambulatory dialysis companies providing emergency water to a hospital during a water contamination crisis
- Hospitals discharging patients to home care partners to clear beds to deal with patient surge during an epidemic
- Behavioral health providers supporting staff and patients of a nursing care center with counseling services following an active shooter/terror attack

in other words

"all hazards" approach

An approach to emergency management that supports a general response capability that is sufficiently nimble to address a range of emergencies of different duration, scale, and cause.

- Hospice grief counselors assisting with psychological first aid following a tornado that destroyed a wing of a hospital and resulted in multiple patient and staff casualties
- Ambulatory surgery center staff assisting a rural hospital emergency department with trauma cases following a train wreck with mass casualties

KEY CONCEPT

Incident Command System

In a crisis, a certain degree of confusion and inefficiency is not uncommon. These are bound to be worse when leadership roles and a hierarchy of command aren't established ahead of time. To prevent this, all inpatient settings are required to choose and implement an incident command system (ICS). This system identifies the people in charge during an emergency and who'll be responsible for carrying out their decisions. Each command center in the system should have an appointed incident commander.

Characteristics of a Successful ICS

The Joint Commission requires inpatient settings to define in their EOPs an ICS that is assimilated into and consistent with the community's command structure. A successful ICS includes the following characteristics:

- **Clarity:** All individuals within the organization must clearly understand their roles and responsibilities.
- **Flexibility:** The structure must be adaptable to a wide variety of situations.
- **Community integration:** The organization's command structure must be coordinated with that of the community responders.

The Federal Emergency Management Agency (FEMA) defines five major ICS management functions as follows:

- **Command:** Sets the emergency response objectives, strategies, and priorities and has overall responsibility for the incident
- **Operations:** Conducts operations to reach the incident objectives; establishes tactics and directs all operational resources
- **Planning:** Supports the incident action planning process by tracking resources, collecting/analyzing information, and maintaining documentation
- **Logistics:** Arranges for resources and needed services to support achievement of the incident objectives
- **Finance and administration:** Monitors costs related to the incident; provides accounting, procurement, time recording, and cost analyses

COLLABORATION: ICS is a standardized structure that allows facilities, staff, procedures, communications, and equipment to operate together and create a coordinated response to an emergency. Leaders, facilities directors, emergency managers, and accreditation professionals, what is your role in the ICS? How does that role coordinate with community responders? How does the ICS help you to work with community response partners representing multiple jurisdictions—municipal, county, state, regional, federal? Talk to each other about expectations. Then clarify them in writing in your EOP.

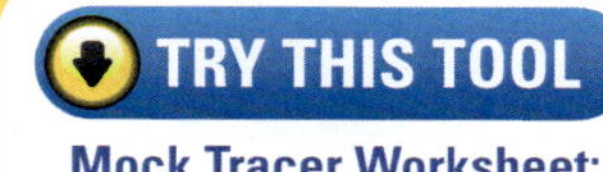

Mock Tracer Worksheet: Incident Command Center
You can use the questions in this mock tracer to trace how (and how well) your incident command center is organized and prepared for emergencies.

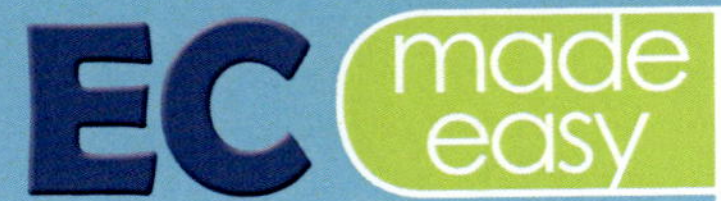

HICS Model

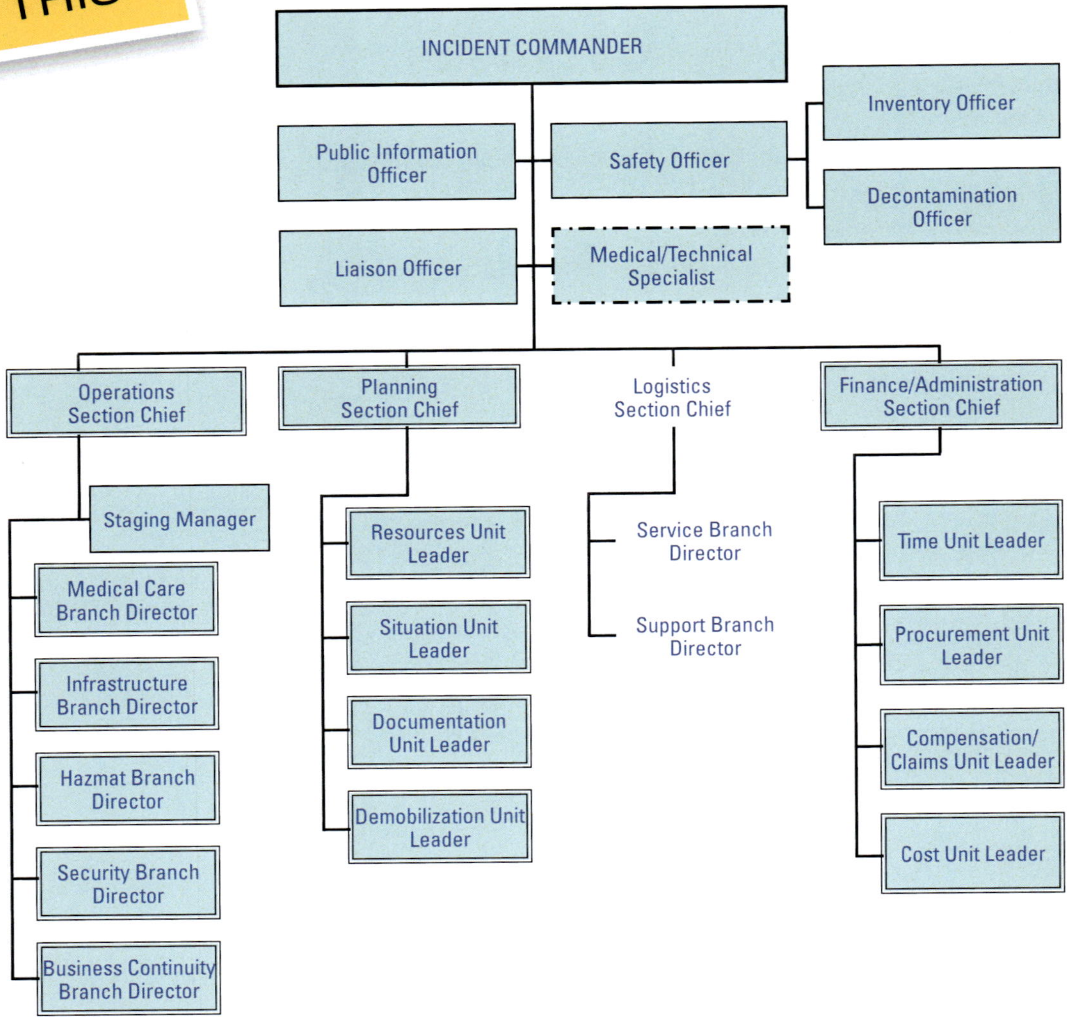

This flowchart shows a common ICS model used by health care organizations: the Hospital Incident Command System (HICS). Although designed for hospitals, it's adaptable to many types of organizations. It presents a temporary organizational structure that allows individuals to be rotated into various roles as time and circumstances dictate. The command staff includes the incident commander, liaison officer, public information officer, safety officer, and medical technical specialist. HICS further defines roles related to operations, planning, logistics, and finance/operations.

KEY CONCEPT

Community Networking

Health care organizations never operate in a vacuum—
especially during an emergency. When you're planning for and
responding to emergencies, community coordination is critical.
In particular, be sure to coordinate with local community
emergency responders (firefighters, police, and emergency
medical technicians), the local public health department, and
any regional or statewide emergency operations entities. Learn
how the local, regional, and statewide emergency operations
command systems function, and, whenever possible, be an
active member in them.

Participation may be through written reviews of community
response plans or e-mail correspondence; in-person meetings
or conference calls; regular participation in health care coalitions, working groups, boards, and committees; educational
events sponsored by the local health department; and regional
training or exercise events sponsored by the state health
department.

It is also important for health care organizations to plan for how
they will support each other during a large-scale emergency.
Organizations should work with their community to plan for
these contingencies. Health care organizations can collaborate
around key issues, such as the following:

- Designation of specific facilities for specific response needs
- Proactive identification and care coordination for vulnerable
  populations
- Crisis risk communication strategies regarding the allocation
  of scarce resources

Communicating needs and vulnerabilities: Most health care
organizations have relationships and understandings with key
components of the community. But it's important to communicate your organization's needs and vulnerabilities to them. Only
then can you determine the community's ability to meet those
needs and accommodate those vulnerabilities.

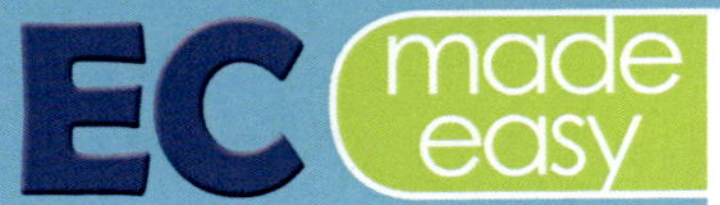

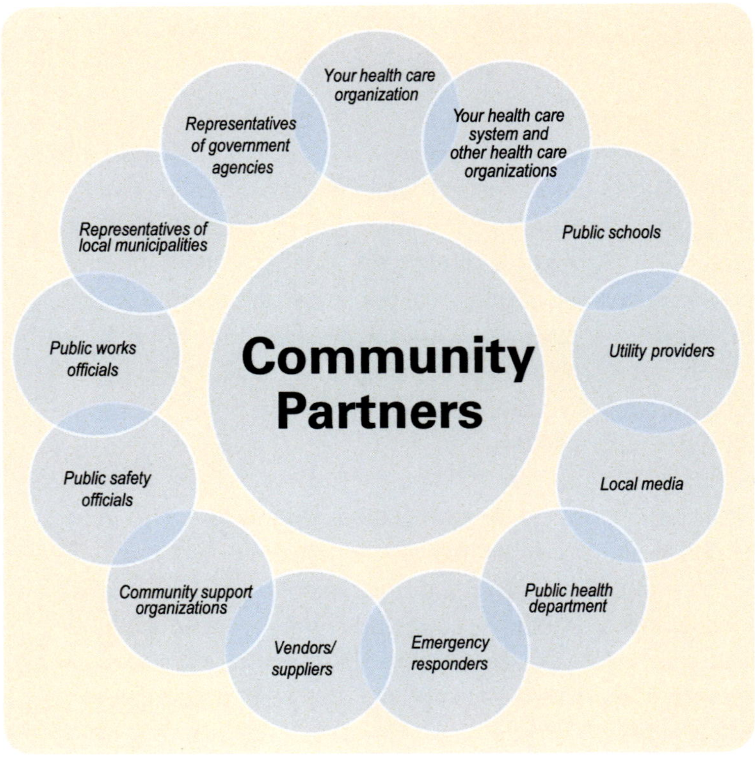

COLLABORATION: To build a relationship with community leaders, you can hold periodic meetings with them. Leaders, demonstrate that you're ready, willing, and able to collaborate by calling and chairing the meetings. Facilities directors, work with your emergency management team to make sure leadership includes key points from your EOP on the agenda. Accreditation professionals, keep your accreditation manual handy to make sure all standards are being addressed in agreements being made.

Emergency Response Exercises

They say practice makes perfect. Although it's unrealistic to expect a perfect response to a crisis, you can and should practice to improve your emergency preparedness. This is usually done by engaging in periodic exercises that stress the limits of your emergency management program and test and assess your EOP. Most importantly, exercises give staff an

in other words

exercise

An activity conducted by an organization to practice, train, and/or drill for emergency events using mock scenarios intended to gauge the effectiveness of the organization's Emergency Operations Plan (EOP).

opportunity to practice their emergency responsibilities under conditions that differ from their usual work routines—different supplies, equipment, team members, patient populations, space, communication technology, time frames. Because no actual emergency adheres to the documented EOP, practice through exercises helps staff respond in a quick and flexible manner through the changing dynamics of emergency response and recovery.

There are many ways in which an organization can evaluate and prepare for likely emergency scenarios and to manage the six critical areas. Seminars, workshops, and tabletop activities can all help familiarize staff with the components, strengths, and gaps in their organization's plan. However, functional exercises provide the most realistic experience for staff to practice their roles and stress the plan to identify weak points and surface opportunities for improvement.

Types of Exercises

Emergency exercises must incorporate likely emergency scenarios that allow the organization to test responses in the six critical areas. Operations-based and full-scale exercises effectively test and validate plans, procedures, and capabilities to respond to emergencies; clarify roles and responsibilities of staff and response partners; and identify resource (staff, supplies, space) and communication gaps:

- Operations-based exercises validate an organization's response plans, staff roles, resources, care processes, and critical infrastructure capabilities.
- Full-scale exercises involve multiple first responders and community agencies, and identify strengths and weaknesses in coordinating linkages for patient care and other emergency response capabilities across response partners.

Required Exercises

The Joint Commission requires most organizations to conduct emergency management exercises twice a year. That applies if your organization offers emergency services or is designated by your community as a disaster-receiving station. If that's not the case, you just need to do them once per year.

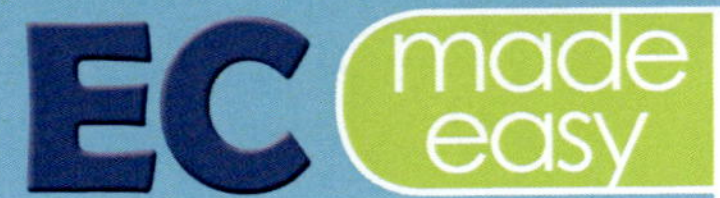

Some exceptions and clarifications: You should check your manual, but for most settings, these exceptions and clarifications apply:

- **Actual emergencies:** If you activated your EOP for an actual emergency, that can take the place of an exercise.
- **Specific tests:** If you have to do two exercises annually, at least one of your tests for each site has to involve the following:
  - *An external disaster that causes an influx of patients:* The patients can be represented by community members who have volunteered to portray disaster victims and/or simulated patients (often represented by paper forms). These mock patients must be triaged, put on gurneys or in wheelchairs, and transported through the system as if they were actual victims.
  - *An escalating event in which the community is unable to support the organization:* This, of course, tests the resources of the organization and its ability to ramp up responses. An example is exercising for a tornado that hits the facility, cuts off the power, and levels the emergency department.
  - *Participation in a communitywide exercise:* Only organizations with a defined role in a community response plan need to have one of these exercises represented in the two per year.
- **Single exercise:** Behavioral health care, home care, and office-based surgery settings are required to conduct only one emergency exercise (or one activation of the emergency plan in response to an actual emergency) each year.
- **Tabletop exercises:** Unless you're accredited under the Home Care Accreditation Program, tabletop exercises don't fulfill the emergency exercise requirement. Home care organizations can use a tabletop exercise to fulfill this requirement—if the organization and the tabletop exercise design meet specific criteria defined in the accreditation manual.

Evaluating the Exercises

The Joint Commission requires you to evaluate each emergency exercise based on its relationship to the risks prioritized in the HVA, and the scope and procedures defined in the EOP.

Useful evaluations: You want to make sure your evaluations are accurate and complete and informative—that is, useful. So gather data during the exercises and document everything well immediately afterward. Here are some general guidelines:

- **Observing:** Designate observers to monitor the required critical areas of emergency response and take notes on what went well—and what could/should have been done better. Photos and video can be useful tools for documenting observations.
- **Quantifying:** Identify areas of strength and weakness via a written critique that can be used to improve the EOP. Quantify the critique by scoring the actions undertaken in each of the required critical areas of response.
- **Sharing:** Share the critique with everyone in the organization and solicit feedback on improvements. Then provide feedback on which feedback was incorporated and why.
- **Comparing:** Compare current critiques to past critiques to identify areas that seem to resist improvement and focus on those for your next exercise.

KEY CONCEPT

Evacuation

The devastating damage caused by the super tornado that hit Joplin, Missouri, in 2011 and the extended power outages in New York City caused by Hurricane Sandy in 2012 resulted in a rare but serious occurrence: the forced evacuation of area hospitals. Evacuation for many facilities is a major endeavor, so you have to be well prepared for it with careful planning.

Evacuation Time Frame

Joint Commission standards require a health care organization to set specific criteria that outline the time frame the organization is able to stay open during an emergency. Part of that decision depends on your access to supplies, staffing, and safe, appropriate space that allow you to sustain independent

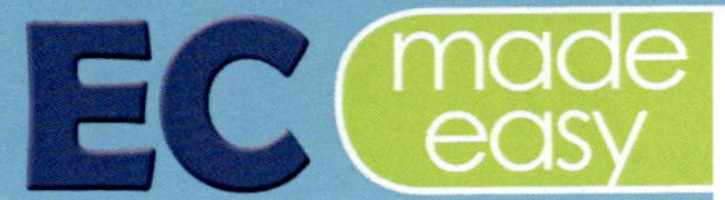

operations for 96 hours. If remaining open for at least 96 hours isn't possible, you should have contingency plans that may include limiting services, conserving resources, and, if the situation demands, evacuating.

Evacuation Process

Safe evacuation requires careful advance planning. Here are the key questions to answer as you define an evacuation process to follow:

- What's the time frame you've committed to staying open before evacuating?
- Who has the authority to call an evacuation?
- Does everyone know that this person has that authority?
- What are the indicators that trigger the decision to evacuate?
- Which patients will be evacuated first?
- What are the precise steps of the evacuation?
- What are the escape routes for horizontal and vertical evacuation (*see* Chapter 7)?
- What's the destination or alternative care site(s) for evacuated patients?
- Who are the external response partners required to support the organization's evacuation procedures? When and how will they be notified of the need to evacuate?
- How will communication between sending organizations, receiving organizations, and other partners supporting evacuation be ensured?
- How will transportation and tracking of patients and equipment be handled during/after evacuation?
- What patient medications and medical records will be needed during/after evacuation?
- What medical equipment will be needed during/after evacuation?
- What staff will need to accompany evacuating patients?
- How will patient location and communication with patient families be tracked and managed?

Don't forget to drill for it: And then, of course, drill the evacuation plan to determine if you have missed anything. You may even want to consider a mock evacuation with volunteer "patients" evacuated to a location in your community and/or outside your community as part of the drill.

KEY CONCEPT

Cyber Emergencies

Cyber, at its simplest, refers to communication over a computer network (internal networks, servers, Internet, cloud).

Routine and advanced health care services are delivered with increasing efficiency, quality, and connectivity across all settings. Examples to consider include the following:

- Electronic health and medication records
- Patient monitoring systems such as telemetry and fetal monitoring
- Medical devices and equipment such as infusion pumps and infant locator systems
- Telemedicine services
- Automated dispensing cabinets
- Ancillary services such as laboratory, radiology, and pharmacy
- Environmental control systems
- Financial and personally identifiable information

Processes for responding to the risk or occurrence of a cyber emergency are complex and rapidly evolving; going beyond issues of access to and confidentiality of electronic health records to the computers, networks, programs, data, and devices that are used in the daily delivery of key health care services.

Cyber Protection

Cyber emergencies occur more and more often. Organizations need to increase preparedness for cyber emergencies that could impact patient care, treatment, or service. Cyber emergencies can take many forms, but the most disruptive to patient care are related to catastrophic system failures or malicious attacks. Organizations must always plan for managing interruptions to information processes, and working with information technology (IT) professionals in your organization is critical to responding to and recovering from cyber emergencies. Risks to information systems, devices, equipment, and technologies that directly impact patient care can be identified, prioritized for preparedness through the HVA, addressed through emergency management planning, and followed up on when identified as opportunities for improvement.

Framework for Preparedness

Cyber emergencies that impact patient care can be managed following a similar framework as for utilities management (*see* Chapter 6), infection prevention and control (*see* Chapter 3), and emergency management (discussed in this chapter):

- Risk awareness
  - Conduct an HVA
- Incident detection
  - Identify that an incident has occurred
- Incident response
  - Repair
  - Recovery
  - Remediate

COLLABORATION: In the typical health care organization, IT is no longer just a department or a lone technician; it is a core utility that supports the functional infrastructure of the organization, as interconnected as electricity. Emergency managers, involve your IT professional or department in emergency management planning to help identify risks that would not be obvious if they were not at the planning table. Your IT staff can help your EM team develop contingency plans if key patient care systems (such as electronic medical records, radiology, laboratory, pharmacy, and telemedicine services) are disabled by a cyber emergency.

TOOLS OF THE TRADE

- Sample Emergency Operations Plan Contents
- 96-Hour Operational Impact Chart
- Emergency Response Staff Training Checklist
- Mock Tracer Worksheet: Incident Command Center

CHAPTER 9

Construction

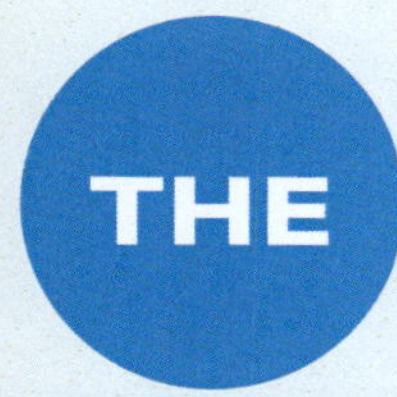

"Pardon our dust" is more than a popular construction sign slogan. It's also a reminder to patients, visitors, and staff that demolition, renovation, and construction at a health care facility can be messy and disruptive. When not well planned and managed, construction projects can even lead to safety problems: diminished air quality, pervasive noise and vibration, dispersed contaminants, and disruption of essential services. Creating a high-quality facility that's built to flex into the future requires your organization to thoroughly prepare for and address the many issues surrounding construction. Primary among those activities are thorough planning and design and risk reduction.

KEY CONCEPTS

- Planning and Design
- Managing Construction Risks
- Commissioning

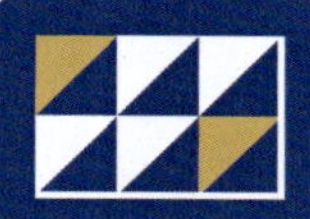

THE MANUAL
Following are the relevant Joint Commission *Comprehensive Accreditation Manual (CAM)* chapters:

- Environment of Care (EC)
- Emergency Management (EM)
- Leadership (LD)
- Infection Prevention and Control (IC)
- Life Safety (LS)

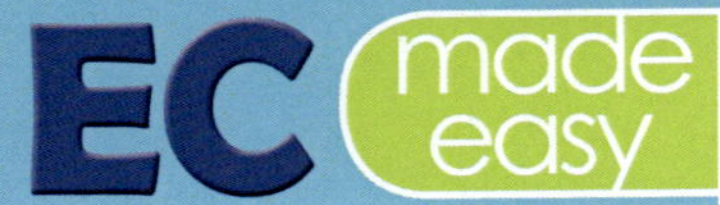

Planning and Design

You may envision your organization's future as one that involves expanding and enhancing services. If you do, that may entail expanding and enhancing your physical structures. To make those visions reality, you need to understand the basics of construction planning and design. Planning and design occur at the beginning of any construction project and are interwoven efforts.

Types of Planning

Planning a construction project is like preparing for a long trip: You need to know why you're traveling, how you're going, who's going with you, and who you'll meet at each key stopping point. You need contingency plans, time, and money. The planning phase involves two types of planning:

- **Master planning:** This is the conceptual type of planning, which entails the following:
  - Outlining goals, strategies, and actions for the future of the facility
  - Considering strategic planning approaches to meet program needs
  - Thinking about projected future growth
- **Predesign:** This is the discovery type of planning that occurs prior to actual design and construction, but usually after some funding is obtained. It involves planning for a specific building project and includes these actions:
  - Outlining project objectives and challenges
  - Conducting studies to determine the following for the project:
    - Space requirements
    - Opportunities and limitations of the site
    - Expected cost vs. the budget

What type of planning happens when: Depending on the size of the structure and the scope of the construction project, you may do both types of planning separately. Or you might combine them into one planning process. Either way, for any predesign planning, you need to take into account concepts considered during master planning.

in other words

master planning

A conceptual process that determines the building needs and plans for an organization over time and involves outlining the goals, strategies, and actions that will carry a facility far into its future.

predesign

The discovery phase of a specific construction project, usually after some funding but before design and construction, that involves outlining project objectives and challenges and conducting studies to examine issues related to space requirements, the site, and the budget.

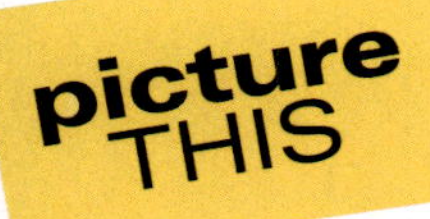

Phases of a Construction Project

Any time you embark on a construction project (especially a large-scale one) it can be helpful to reduce that project to small, easy-to-manage parts. Most building projects can be organized into distinct phases. Although some phases can overlap, they're usually implemented sequentially. The phases shown here provide a framework for structuring a building project.

Phase 1. Planning
This includes "blue sky" ("wish list") considerations, master planning, and predesign efforts.

Phase 2. Schematic design
This involves drawing a rough outline of the project, including preliminary room layout, structure, and scope.

Phase 3. Design and development
This includes adding details to the design, such as equipment, fixtures, furniture location, and decor.

Phase 4. Construction documentation
This requires converting the design into a template for contractors to use to estimate costs, identify issues, and plan construction activities. At this point, organizations will discuss contract conditions.

Phase 5. Construction
This is the phase in which the structure or facility is actually built.

Phase 6. Commissioning
This encompasses making sure that all specifications are met and that all systems, components, equipment, and so forth are fully operational. This activity should happen throughout the project to ensure a good project that can be completed through final certifications.

Phase 7. Occupancy
This involves moving into the space and closing out the project.

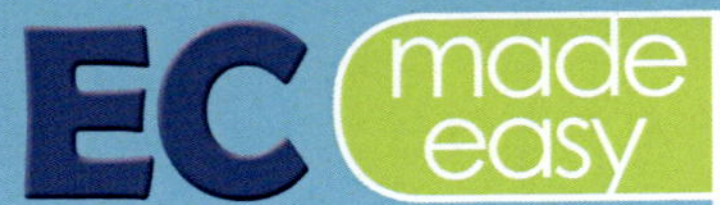

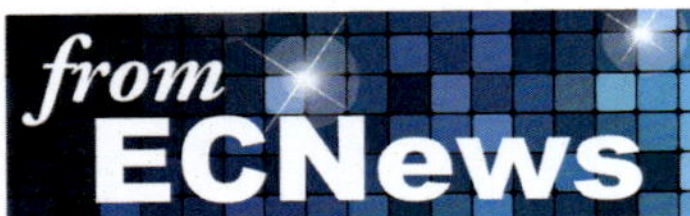

Construction Needs Analysis

One activity to consider during the data collection process is a needs analysis. This detailed assessment for each department or service looks at current capacity, projected needs, and strategic goals for the particular department or service. For example, as part of a needs assessment for a maternity unit, your organization may examine population projections of women ages 15 to 44, including historical and projected fertility rates by geographic area. Similarly, in assessing the needs of the surgical service, your organization may examine the impact of managed care and estimate what the population-based surgical procedure rate will be in the future.

Marketing studies and demographic analyses are often part of a needs analysis. These types of research can help your organization get information on a variety of topics, including the following:

- Service areas
- The payer mix of constituents
- Community perceptions of the facility and a potential construction project
- Appropriate location of a new facility
- Potential lost revenue due to a construction project or relocation of a facility
- The presence and impact of competition

—excerpted from "It All Starts with a Good Plan: Master Planning Creates a Road Map for Change," *Environment of Care® News,* February 2011

Steps in the Planning Phase

The planning phase of a construction project should be an organized process of specific tasks, benchmarks, and checkpoints. It should also be an interactive process involving an interdisciplinary team. Important steps in this process include the following:

- **Step 1 — Analyzing project needs:** Your organization may need to research and/or perform a needs analysis to evaluate various project needs, including these:
  - Whether to renovate or build new (*see* the Key Concept "Managing Construction Risks" on page 175)
  - Possible locations for any proposed new building sites
  - Needs of the organization's service areas
  - How to address community perceptions of the project
- **Step 2 — Assembling the project team:** In addition to a team leader (who may be the construction leader on the facilities staff), your team will ideally include the following people:
  - Administrative and clinical leaders
  - Accreditation and other regulatory professionals (including the safety officer)
  - Representatives of various departments and programs—including finance and infection prevention and control
  - External project consultants (architects, engineers, contractors)
  - Community representatives
- **Step 3 — Gathering project data:** A construction project planning team makes a lot of decisions based on a lot of data. For example, the team uses data about the following:
  - Operational structures
  - Existing services
  - Property boundaries and features
  - Existing facilities on the property
- **Step 4 — Devising a construction project plan:** This plan should cover many important activities, including the following:
  - Project phasing and scheduling
  - Existing space measurements and the project's general goal for spatial/physical organization (*see* the sidebar "A Detailed Space Program" on page 170)

- Long- and short-term cost-benefits of the specific project and related projects
- Future growth projections

- **Step 5 — Determining a budget:** This is a core step, so all cost factors need consideration, not just construction costs. A good budget includes costs related to the following:

  - Land
  - Construction
  - Fees
  - Interest
  - Start-up
  - Moving
  - Equipment
  - Furnishings
  - Contingencies

- **Step 6 — Creating and phasing in the master plan:** The master plan is the final construction project plan that incorporates all the planning and design objectives and targeted concerns. Many organizations consider it a living document that the team revises, revisits, and updates regularly.

- **Step 7 — Securing a certificate of need (CON):** This involves justifying to the state why the construction project is necessary. Some states require this; others don't. The process allows states to provide a balance of services across health care organizations and ensures that each one is adequately serving its community. If your state requires one, have a preliminary review with CON hearing staff early in the planning process and allow extra time in the schedule for the CON hearing process. You might consider retaining a CON consultant to assist you in this process.

- **Step 8 — Documenting and summarizing the master plan:** Text, tables, drawings, and other parts of your master plan should be documented in a way that makes them easy to use, share, and store. You might put the master plan into a book or binder or other organization document. This document should contain up front an executive summary that highlights key goals, facts, issues, assumptions, needs, and master planning concepts.

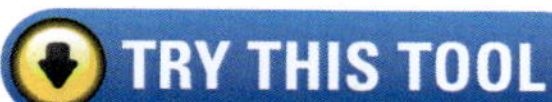

Construction Project Cost Worksheet
Your organization can use this worksheet to record and monitor typical expenses related to a health care construction project.

in other words

master plan
The final construction plan that incorporates all the planning and design objectives and targeted concerns.

smart questions:

For any current/recent construction projects, who is/was part of your project team?

COLLABORATION: Two of the main advantages of collaboration in construction planning and design are the involvement of various experts and the streamlining of approvals. Accreditation professionals, you need to lend your knowledge of relevant Joint Commission requirements for the project. That includes those that impact compliance with standards related to operations in the finished structure. Leaders, you can help the project in many ways, but especially by granting approvals in a timely manner to avoid delays. Facilities directors and construction leaders, make sure that leaders have the information needed to do that by keeping careful records and planning within established budgets. If the project involves renovation or expansion of an existing facility, interim life safety measures (ILSMs) may also need to be devised, which will require your expertise.

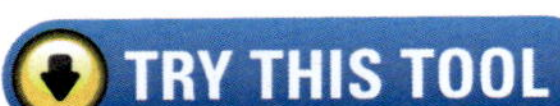

Room Data Sheet
This form can be used in preparing your detailed space program.

A Detailed Space Program

Before budgeting for a construction project, you need to outline the space you need to meet your goals and objectives. This involves estimating key patient care spaces (patient beds, exam rooms, operating rooms) as well as other space elements to support them. This is typically known as a detailed space program.

You can create a detailed space program by using likely scenarios and forecasted workloads. This is done through working sessions with departmental representatives, tours of similar facilities, and examples from previous projects.

A Summary List

A detailed space program usually involves a summary list that identifies department, building, and project area subtotals and totals. The list should also include a room-by-room space list, organized by department, functional area, or physical component of the building or project. At a minimum, this list should identify the name, number, and size of every room, space, area, and department to be included in the project.

A Narrative Description

Frequently, a narrative description is provided for all key spaces. It identifies how the size and character of each space is determined. This detailed information may also be recorded on separate forms called room data sheets, which are developed for each room.

Build or Renovate?

During planning for major construction projects, you'll probably evaluate whether to build new facilities or renovate existing ones. In some cases, you can renovate and convert existing space for less money than you can build new space. Often, though, renovation costs may exceed construction costs due to things like unforeseen conditions, phasing, scheduling, and logistical complexities.

Renovation viability: A wide variety of conditions will determine the viability of renovation, including the following:
- Amount, type, and location of space available for renovation
- Mechanical and electrical system limitations
- Ability to work within the existing building's boundaries
- Location of columns and structural walls
- Location of vertical penetrations (openings), such as mechanical shafts, elevators, and fire stairs
- Location of staging area—either close in proximity or some distance away from the site
- Temporary parking for visitors, patients, staff, and contractors
- Abatement of hazards (such as asbestos in older buildings)

Renovation issues: Some issues to consider when deciding whether renovation is the best option are the following:
- **Functionality:** How will the space function to support the mission of the organization and its role in the community? How large is the discrepancy between the current space and the desired functionality?
- **Adaptability:** How can the space be adapted for the desired use? How much will it cost to adapt? What systems or services will be compromised by the renovation?
- **State of the facility:** Can the infrastructure support the new technology? Will the utility systems or communication/technology infrastructure need upgrading or expanding to meet the demands of the new space and can it be? What hidden costs might arise, such as removal of hazardous materials such as asbestos or lead?

- **Ability to meet current requirements:** Will all systems meet current fire and safety code requirements for the new space, or will they need updating? Will the renovation affect the organization's ability to meet accreditation standards? To meet other laws and regulations (*see* the sidebar "Americans with Disabilities Act (ADA)" below)?
- **Physical age:** How much useful life is left in the major construction elements of the facility? Will they need replacement? Is it cost-effective to replace aging utility systems with new, more efficient versions?
- **Future-proofing ability:** How long will it be before the renovation needs updating? How long for new construction?
- **Cost of downtime:** Will the project deter patients from using the facility? Will temporary alternative facilities be needed?
- **Hybrid approach:** Can the project renovate some of the existing elements and replace others?

Americans with Disabilities Act (ADA)

The Americans with Disabilities Act (ADA), signed into law in 1990, prohibits discrimination against people with disabilities. This means that health care facilities are required to be readily accessible to and usable by individuals with disabilities. And they must also reduce safety risks for those individuals. For example, a wheelchair-accessible bathroom stall should have a grab bar installed to prevent falls and injuries.

ADA Accessibility Guidelines

Medical facilities must ensure that disabled individuals, including those with mobility and vision impairments, can get around safely. Newly constructed offices and buildings, along with those that have undergone renovations or major modifications, should be constructed or remodeled in compliance with the ADA accessibility guidelines. These guidelines provide detailed specifications on parking, ramps, door widths, restroom facilities, and other features that affect accessibility. Equipment and furniture selection should also include consideration of the needs of individuals who use wheelchairs and scooters or who have difficulty moving around.

Guidelines influence: The architectural principles of universal design ensure that facilities, products, and services are usable by all people. Through application of those principles, the ADA's parameters greatly influence the design, construction, and operation of health care buildings and equipment.

Guidelines compliance: Joint Commission standards require compliance with all local, state, and federal laws and regulations, including the ADA. In addition, state and local building code authorities typically require compliance with the ADA.

Key Considerations for the Long Term

Aging health care facilities pose critical problems all over the country, in part because many were designed and constructed without realizing how long they might have to last and how flexible they'd need to be. While engaged in planning and design, you need to keep in mind some key considerations to ensure a structure that's safe and effective over the long term—which may be for many decades. These issues include the following:

- **Needs of the community:** Is there a large geriatric population in the community? Will that population grow during the life of the structure? What about the pediatric population? Is it growing or shrinking? Should the organization plan special spaces for these populations and others?
- **Environmental matters:** How is the building sited, or situated on the proposed parcel of land? Is the location vulnerable to possible shifts in the land or area waterways? What building materials are planned? How long will they last in your current climate? In a changed climate? What are the environmental concerns for waste disposal in your area? For water and energy use—now and in the future?
- **Technology innovations:** Is the facility designed to accommodate recent technological innovations? Can it "flex into the future" to adapt to new ones?
- **Efficiency and sustainability:** Is the structure efficient and sustainable? Is its design flexible enough to respond to changing needs without requiring major structural adjustments?

COLLABORATION: The most encompassing standards regarding facility design are those in the "Leadership" (LD) chapter of the accreditation manual. That chapter provides broad statements about responsibility and accountability. But the intent goes deep and requires very specific outcomes. Leaders, you're responsible for analyzing and developing programs that meet the community's needs. You're accountable to the community for the results of those programs. That means you need to collaborate with community leaders from day 1 of any construction project.

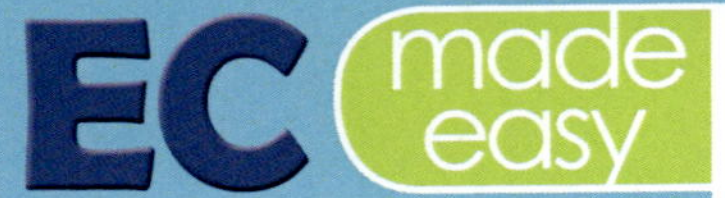

Evidence-Based Design

In the environment of care, as in clinical care, evidence-based practices (or best practices) offer proven examples and guidelines to follow. Evidence-based design (EBD) practices help you to create facilities that enhance patient safety, help patients recover faster, and help staff perform better. Design principles included in EBD address the following:

- Building private rooms
- Reducing noise levels
- Incorporating nature into building designs
- Improving air quality
- Implementing natural and artificial light sources
- Employing a decentralized design that allows staff to work closer to patients

Healing design: Many aspects of EBD (natural light, noise reduction, access to nature) are important components of a healing environment for patients. Other aspects of facility design that promote healing include art, music, social interaction areas, noninstitutional design, and age-appropriate design.

Required Design Criteria

Whether you're going for modern or traditional design, taking a state-of-the art approach, or being conservative, you must abide by regulations. The Joint Commission requires you to use one or more of the following design criteria when planning new or renovated facilities:

- State rules and regulations
- The Facility Guidelines Institute's 2014 *Guidelines for Hospitals and Outpatient Facilities*
- Other reputable standards and guidelines that provide equivalent design criteria

Designing for Laboratories and Pharmacies

Laboratories and pharmacies are vital components of many health care facilities. The needs of laboratories and pharmacies are distinctly different, however, from those of construction projects that deal mainly with patient care and support rooms. If a construction or renovation project includes a laboratory or pharmacy, involve relevant management early and throughout the planning and design phases to avoid costly changes later.

KEY CONCEPT

Managing Construction Risks

At least one person in your organization has been given the responsibility of risk management in the environment of care (*see* Chapter 1). But everyone involved in a construction project should be ready to provide input to help manage risks. Some risks may be present during construction only. Others are potential risks in finished structures that need to be addressed during planning and design.

Construction Risks in Environment of Care Areas

Throughout this book, you've learned about various areas of the environment of care. While planning and designing any construction project, give careful thought to these areas:

- **Safety:** It might be the sudden collapse of a scaffold on a worker. It might be the slow release of toxic fumes into a patient care area in a new wing. You have to prepare for worst-case scenarios and ensure that all building occupants are safe at all times, including contracted construction workers (*see* Chapter 3).
- **Security:** Any or all of the following security issues should be kept in mind during planning and design (*see* Chapter 4):
  - Selecting appropriate alarm systems, security cameras, and panic buttons
  - Creating floor layouts that enhance security
  - Designing emergency departments that control access to waiting, triage, and treatment areas
  - Incorporating features to help prevent theft, abduction, and suicide
- **Hazardous materials and waste:** You should design layouts and install equipment and furnishings that help prevent exposure to hazardous materials and waste—including infectious waste (*see* Chapter 5 and page 76). Consider the following:
  - Placing of hand sinks, alcohol-based hand rub dispensers, and negative-pressure rooms
  - Engineering the heating, ventilating, and air-conditioning (HVAC) system effectively
  - Minimizing use of carpet, which can hold and foster growth of harmful fungi and bacteria

- Installing effective water systems
- Choosing appropriate, nonhazardous wall sealants, finishes, and materials
- Hazardous materials present *during* construction (explained later in this chapter)

- **Medical equipment and utility systems:** Operation of medical equipment and utility systems may be affected during construction and could be the cause of serious failures or accidents (*see* Chapter 6). Plans for new space should also incorporate safe storage and use of these vital components. Equipment planning is an essential and time-critical element of health facility planning and development. Selection of equipment, such as an x-ray machine or PET scanner, will often affect the size and layout of a space. To determine the equipment space and design needs, a preliminary equipment list should be developed as part of the planning process.

- **Fire safety and life safety:** Joint Commission standards mandate that health care facilities, whether newly constructed, renovated, or existing, abide by the *Life Safety Code*,* which helps organizations protect patients, staff, and visitors from threats posed by fire (*see* Chapter 7). There are two ways you need to comply with the *Life Safety Code* during the building process:
  - When you plan and design a building, you must ensure that the building meets the requirements outlined by the *Life Safety Code*.
  - During construction, you must ensure that compliance is maintained during the construction process by developing interim life safety measures (ILSMs) (*see* the sidebar "ILSMs During Construction" on page 177).

- **Emergency management:** Don't forget to consider emergency management issues (*see* Chapter 8) during planning and design of new spaces, as well as how such issues might be affected during construction. These include parking, patient flow through the facility, and how to convert spaces into triage, patient care, or holding areas.

ILSMs During Construction

The Joint Commission's Life Safety (LS) standards require you to comply with the *Life Safety Code®*, which helps protect facility occupants from smoke and fire. But during construction and renovation, you may have a life safety deficiency that can't be fixed right away. What do you do? You can put appropriate interim life safety measures (ILSMs) into effect (also *see* Chapter 7). The 11 measures to choose from, as outlined in the LS standards, include the following:

- **Exits:** Inspect exits in affected areas on a daily basis.
- **Signals and alarms:** Make sure that temporary but equivalent fire alarm and detection systems are in place when a fire system is impaired.
- **Firefighting equipment:** Provide additional extinguishers and other firefighting equipment, which should be adequately and safely stored in the affected area.
- **Construction barriers:** Use temporary construction partitions that are smoke tight and fireproof/fire-resistant.
- **Surveillance:** Boost surveillance of buildings, groups, and equipment, with a special focus on construction areas and storage, excavation, and field offices.
- **Debris:** Lower the building's combustible load by enforcing debris-removal practices.
- **Firefighting equipment training:** Offer additional training to staff on the use of firefighting equipment.
- **Fire drills:** Conduct one additional fire drill per shift per quarter.
- **Inspection and testing:** Inspect and test temporary systems monthly.
- **Education:** Provide education to promote awareness of building deficiencies, construction hazards, and temporary measures implemented to maintain fire safety.
- **Fire safety features training:** Train staff to compensate for impaired structural or compartmental fire safety features.

Preconstruction Risk Assessment

One of the most important aspects of any construction project is the preconstruction risk assessment. The Joint Commission requires you to conduct a preconstruction risk assessment during the construction planning phase. It should identify hazards that could compromise patient care and occupant safety in your facility *during construction itself*. The Facility Guidelines Institute requires a similar assessment that it calls an infection control risk assessment (ICRA).

in other words

preconstruction risk assessment

A risk assessment required before construction projects that addresses the impact of construction on patient care and occupant safety in a facility during construction.

Construction risks to assess: The type of construction affects the degree of the assessment and determines what risk areas should be addressed. Your preconstruction risk assessment should at least consider the impact construction will have on areas like infection control, utilities, and the emergency department. Examples of issues to consider include the following:

- Disruption of essential services
- Discovery of hazardous materials and mold
- Relocation or placement of patients
- Traffic flow (both vehicular and pedestrian)
- Debris cleanup and removal

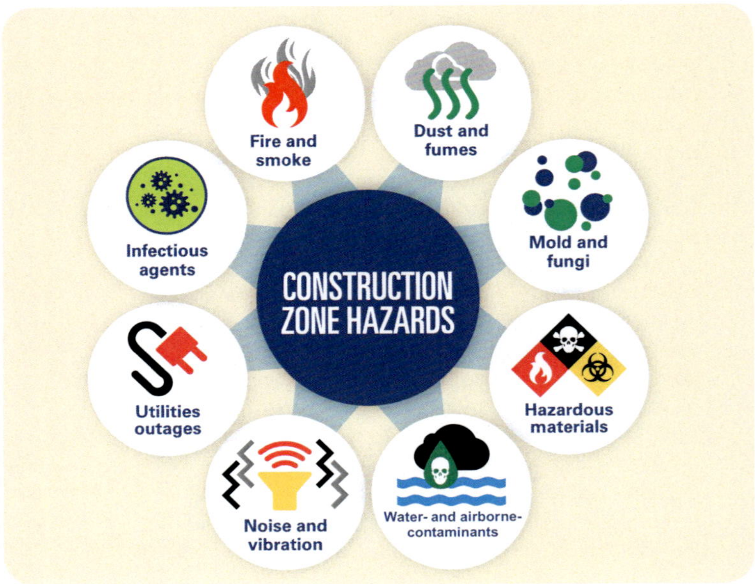

Conducting the preconstruction risk assessment: Suggested steps in conducting a preconstruction risk assessment include the following:

Step 1: Determine the scope of the assessment
Step 2: Pick a team
Step 3: Review applicable guidelines
Step 4: Determine the hazards
Step 5: Respond to the hazards

Using a matrix: Many organizations construct a matrix to make sure each risk has an appropriate response. A matrix typically includes the following ranked categories of information:

- **Activities:** Types of construction project activity (from minor to major)
- **Patients:** Groups of patients affected (from low to high risk)
- **Issues:** Classes of issues involved with the project and related precautions to minimize related risks (from simple to complex)

The patient risk group (choosing the highest risk if there's more than one affected) is then matched to the type of project activity to find the class of precaution to take.

COLLABORATION: A preconstruction risk assessment is most effective when carried out by an interdisciplinary team. This team can include risk managers, experts in facility design, infection control practitioners, safety officers, building engineers, direct care supervisors, and building contractors. Leaders, facilities directors, and accreditation professionals, you'll find collaborating with this team is necessary to understand the scope and depth of safety risks posed by a construction project.

Minimizing Construction Site Risks

To minimize risks in construction sites, your organization and construction crews need to adopt safety strategies. These include the following:

- **Isolation by barriers:** Use barriers to separate the construction area from adjacent areas.
- **Utility system checks:** Make sure that HVAC systems are working properly and test regularly for air and water quality.
- **Proper work equipment and methods:** Require construction workers to be thoroughly trained in safety measures and the special parameters of doing construction in a health care setting. They should know how to use appropriate equipment and methods such as the following:
  - Negative air pressure machines (HEPA [high-efficiency particulate air]–filtered units) to filter and redirect air and vacuums to decrease dust

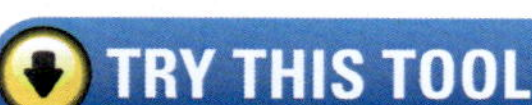

Mock Tracer Worksheet: Construction Site
This worksheet includes questions to ask during a mock tracer for construction site safety, including questions about ILSMs.

- Tacky mats and covered waste containers to contain dust
- Low-emitting products to prevent off-gassing of carcinogens into the air
- Personal protective equipment (PPE) and clothing to protect construction workers (and staff working near the site)
- Working off-hours to reduce impact on building occupants
- **Protective environment (PE) rooms:** Protect patients with compromised immune systems from possible contaminants in the environment by an increased positive pressure airflow from the patient's room to general areas.
- **Signage:** Create and post highly visible construction boards.
- **Traffic control:** Keep construction traffic separate from that of patients, staff, and visitors.

KEY CONCEPT

Commissioning

Imagine being handed the keys to your newly built dream home. You walk in, but the door won't close properly, the heat or air-conditioning doesn't work, and the electricity is dead. This kind of nightmare scenario can happen in new health care facilities, too. That's why you need to make sure to build in a "commissioning" phase in the construction process. Commissioning is a systematic process that verifies, documents, and tests building components and systems to guarantee that they're up to snuff and performing to specifications.

Steps in the Commissioning Phase

The commissioning process typically starts in the design phase and can continue a year or more after the project is finished. The advantages of commissioning are greater efficiency, improved safety, and cost savings realized by avoiding retrofitting, downtime, and unwanted events. Steps involved in commissioning can include the following:

Step 1 — OPR: Draft and fulfill an owner's project requirements (OPR) document.

Step 2 — Documentation: Thoroughly document and review system design, operating sequences, and testing procedures.

---

in other words

construction boards

Customizable signage placed in and around a health care facility during construction to communicate important information to staff, patients, and visitors about disruptions, noise levels, and other safety issues.

commissioning

A series of activities before taking ownership of a building, project, or renovation, in which an organization makes sure that all specifications are met and that all systems, components, equipment, and such are fully operational.

owner's project requirements (OPR)

A living document used throughout the commissioning process that defines how the owner wants the building to operate and function. This document, a narrative description used to develop the basis of the design by the design team, includes the owner's wish list and specifications for the project.

Step 3 — Verification and monitoring: Verify and monitor system performance based on tests and measurements.

Step 4 — Operations training: Train building operations staff on how to operate and maintain the facility (sometimes referred to as "clinical commissioning").

Step 5 — Leadership transfer: Turn the facility over to organization leadership.

TOOLS OF THE TRADE

- Construction Project Cost Worksheet
- Room Data Sheet
- Mock Tracer Worksheet: Construction Site

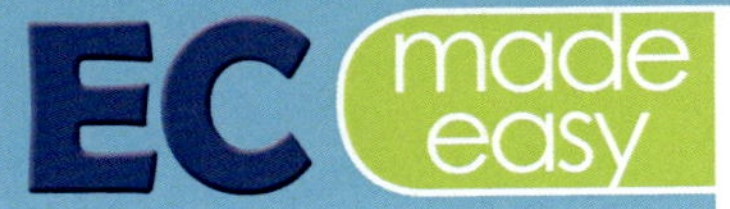

Chapter 10

The EC Survey

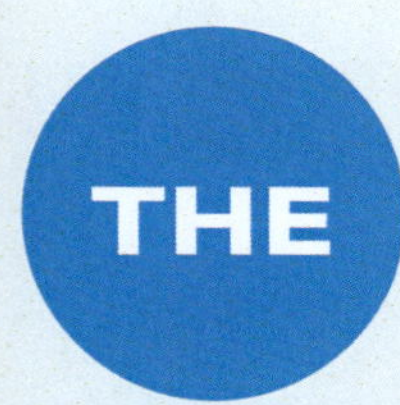

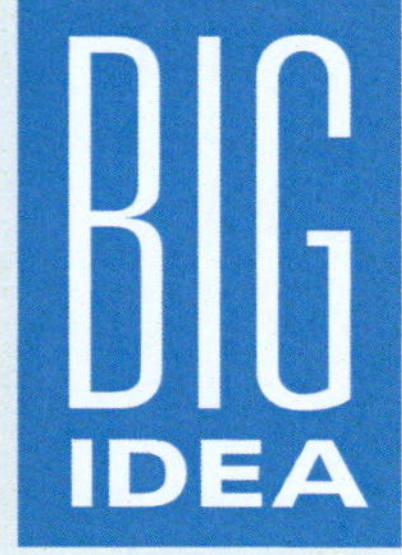

A Joint Commission survey is about much more than getting an accreditation certificate—it's a process that supports the overall goal of a consistently high level of patient safety and quality of care, treatment, and services. The entire Joint Commission accreditation system is designed to keep that goal a conscious priority at every level of an organization. The environment of care (EC) gets special attention during a survey, with dedicated sessions and activities such as tracers and tours.

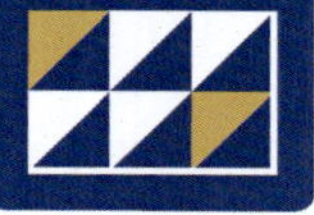

THE MANUAL

Following is the relevant Joint Commission *Comprehensive Accreditation Manual* (*CAM*) chapter:

- The Accreditation Process (ACC)

KEY CONCEPTS

- The On-Site Survey Process
- The Survey Analysis for Evaluating Risk™ (SAFER™) Matrix
- After the Survey
- Continuous Compliance

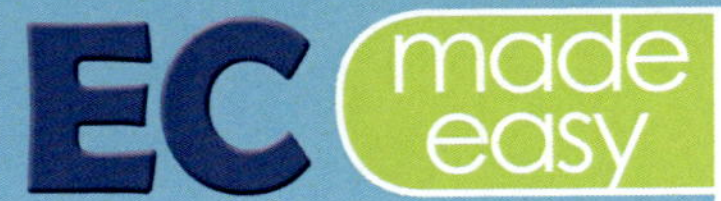

The On-Site Survey Process

Observe processes, review documents, ask questions, take notes, assess compliance, offer strategies, provide feedback, and create reports. That's what accreditation professionals do on a daily basis to help maintain compliance with Joint Commission standards. And that's pretty much what Joint Commission surveyors do during an on-site survey.

Types of surveys: Just what will *your* survey be like? Well, that depends on your organization, which accreditation program it will be surveyed under, and other factors. You may experience several different types of surveys. Or you may have a single two-day survey and be done. The various types of surveys are summarized in "The Accreditation Process" (ACC) chapter of your *Comprehensive Accreditation Manual* (*CAM*).

Frequency of surveys: Except in very specific circumstances, every accredited organization must undergo an on-site survey between 18 and 36 months after its last full survey. (If you're accredited under the Laboratory Accreditation Program, the time frame is shortened to 24 months.) The survey could come at any time during this span, which encourages your organization to maintain consistent compliance and survey readiness.

The physical environment portion of the survey: The full on-site survey addresses the physical environment in several ways, some of which are common to other parts of the survey—with slight variations. For example, the *Life Safety Code*®* surveyor briefly explains the structure and content of the survey. In turn, you briefly explain your organization's structures, mission, and other big-picture information related to the physical environment. Other parts of the survey will be specific to the environment of care, but any surveyor may address environment of care–related issues they observe (*see* page 189).

Documentation

The surveyor should be provided with all requested information and documentation. This information is evaluated on its own merits and used throughout the survey as reference and also to create tracers (*see* page 186) and conduct other survey activities.

- **Requested EC documents:** Commonly requested documents for the environment of care include the following:
  - Minutes from the EC committee meetings for the previous 12 months (*see* Chapter 1)
  - Annual evaluations of the EC management plans (*see* Chapter 2)
  - Life safety drawings (*see* Chapter 7)
  - Interim life safety measures (ILSMs) policy (*see* Chapters 7 and 9)
  - Written fire response plan (*see* Chapter 7)
  - Documentation of inspection, testing, and maintenance for medical equipment and utility components (*see* Chapter 6) and life safety equipment (*see* Chapter 7)
  - Emergency management (EM) documents, such as the Emergency Operations Plan (EOP) and the hazard vulnerability analysis (HVA) (*see* Chapter 8)
- **Required written documentation:** Additional documents may be requested as well. Documentation identified in a standard or element of performance (EP) labeled with the **D** icon should be provided to surveyors on request during any part of the survey. You can refer to the "Required Written Documentation" (RWD) chapter in the *CAMs* or try using the documentation filter available in the E-dition®, the electronic version of the *CAMs*. There is also a general list in the *Accreditation Survey Activity Guide for Health Care Organizations*, which is kept updated on your organization's *Joint Commission Connect™* extranet site.

Where are your EC documents stored so that they're available for surveyors?

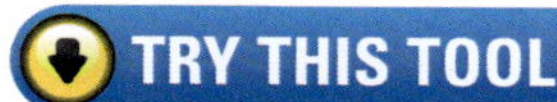

Required EC Documentation Checklist
Use this checklist to guide your EC documentation as well as to check that all of the required documentation is in your survey binder, ready if your surveyor requests it.

in other words

required written documentation (RWD)
A procedure, policy, plan, license, or other piece of written information that goes beyond that included in a medical record and is necessary for accreditation compliance. The documentation can be on paper or in an electronic format.

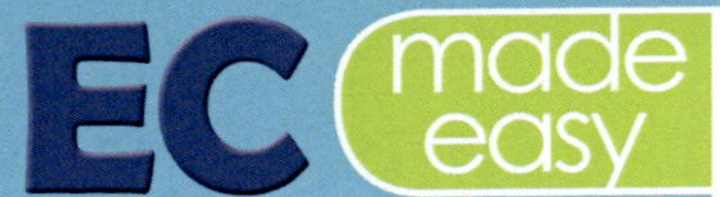

in other words

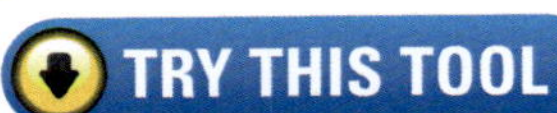

tracer

A tool used by surveyors to analyze an organization's systems by following or "tracing" an individual patient through the care process.

⬇ TRY THIS TOOL

Tracer Questions and the Mock Tracer Form
This document provides a digital mock tracer form you may want to try for your mock tracers, and provides directions on how to use it.

Environment of Care Tracers

A tracer is a tool used to follow or "trace" a patient through his or her process of care. Tracers are the primary tool used by surveyors for on-site surveys. Some tracers focus on the experience of the patient and how the various aspects of an organization interact to meet the patient's needs and maintain safety. Others examine a specific program or system in the organization.

Environment of care tracers: The environment of care is either integrated as part of patient or system tracers or a part of the environment of care/emergency management system session during a survey. EC tracers examine organization systems and processes related to the physical environment, emergency management, and life safety. An EC tracer is often triggered by something a surveyor observes during a patient tracer; for example, surveyors may notice environment-based risks associated with a patient and the staff providing care, treatment, or services to that person.

High-risk tracers: During any type of tracer, a surveyor may see specific high-risk areas that require a more in-depth look. At that point, the surveyor may decide to conduct an additional tracer, one that allows a deeper and more detailed exploration of a particular area, process, or subject. During an on-site survey, tracers will often identify environment of care issues that require a closer look. For example, a surveyor conducting an individual tracer of a patient might notice an employee mishandling hazardous waste, which would spark a follow-up tracer directly related to this important environment of care area. You should also be prepared to participate in tracer activities in other areas that may be related to the physical environment, such as infection prevention and control and clinical areas that may involve medical equipment management.

Mock tracers: You can use tracers the same way surveyors do and for similar purposes by conducting simulated—or mock—tracers in your organization that mimic actual tracers. Mock tracers are helpful in the following ways:
- To engage staff and leadership in accreditation activities, such as regular assessment of compliance with standards

- To help you identify deficiencies so you can address them with interventions and sustain improvements
- To better prepare you for your next on-site survey
- To reduce anxiety about the survey process, which will allow for a more relaxed and beneficial experience

The Environment of Care and Emergency Management Session

The on-site survey includes a special set of activities that relate directly to the EC standards, known as the Environment of Care and Emergency Management Session. (Life Safety [LS] standards are assessed during the *Life Safety Code* Session and Building Assessment.) During this time, the surveyor evaluates your organization's systems and practices for managing environment of care risks. Two primary components make up the EC and EM Session: group discussion and observation.

Group discussion: The group discussion includes organization representatives who can address EC management issues with the surveyor.

- **Discussion participants:** Participants might include the coordinators of safety management activities, the facilities director, and individuals responsible for management of the six EC functional areas (safety, security, hazardous materials and waste, fire safety, medical equipment, and utilities), the chair of the EC Committee, organizational leadership, risk management, patient safety representatives, clinical representatives, support services, and, if applicable, those responsible for the physical environment at remote sites (*see* Chapter 1).
- **Discussion topics:** The surveyor will lead the group in a discussion of each of the six EC functional areas. This session is not intended to be an interview; surveyors would like to listen to the group's discussion of how risk is addressed in the functional areas in the following management processes:
  - *Plan:* What risks have you identified related to this functional area?
  - *Teach:* How do you communicate roles/responsibilities to staff (including contract staff) and volunteers?

- **_Implement:_** What have you done to minimize the impact of risk to patients, visitors, and staff?
- **_Respond:_** What do you do when an incident/failure in one of these functional areas occurs? How, when, and to whom do staff report problems, incidents, and/or failures?
- **_Monitor:_** How do you monitor environment of care performance (both human activities and physical components)? What monitoring activities have taken place within the last 12 months?
- **_Improve:_** Are you currently analyzing any environment of care or emergency management issues? What actions have been taken as a result?

Observation: The observation portion of the EC and EM Session involves exactly that: the surveyor observing how the management processes are put into practice in the "real world" of the organization. This is the tracer portion of the survey (as described earlier). The surveyor considers EC documents reviewed, observations made, and knowledge gained from the group discussion and determines which processes are most likely to cause risk. These processes are then traced as follows:

- **Identifying the point of risk:** The surveyor finds out where the risk is happening. For example, is it the location of a security incident? The place a particular piece of equipment is used?
- **Conducting staff interviews:** The surveyor asks staff about their roles in minimizing that risk and how they respond when it occurs, including reporting afterward.
- **Assessing risk control:** The surveyor evaluates how and how well physical controls operate in minimizing the risk (alarms, contingency plans).
- **Reviewing procedures:** The surveyor goes over all relevant inspection, testing, and maintenance procedures.
- **Conducting further interviews:** The surveyor talks to others who may play a role in responding to an incident or situation.

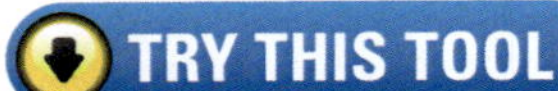

⊙ TRY THIS TOOL

On-Site Survey Readiness Checklist

This checklist is designed to help you prepare for a surveyor's visit to practice the procedures.

Summary discussion: At the end of the EC and EM Session, the surveyor summarizes any potential vulnerabilities for those responsible for managing that process, as well as performs a review of the building assessment. A discussion follows, covering the organizational and staff response to the risk and how existing activities address the potential vulnerabilities.

COLLABORATION: Facilities directors and accreditation professionals, send out an invitation to staff and leaders to find those interested in meeting with you about their experiences in a recent survey. Ask for positive feedback as well as suggestions for improving what went wrong. Solicit volunteers interested in helping with EC survey readiness activities or committee. If your organization doesn't already have one, build a mock tracer program and make sure that EC and EM issues are routinely addressed. Collaboration is vital not only during survey but also leading up to and following it.

The *Life Safety Code* Session

Like the EC and EM Session, there is a part of the on-site survey that focuses on Life Safety (LS) standards (*see* Chapter 7). The *Life Safety Code* Session and Building Assessment focuses on the following:

- Your process for designing and maintaining buildings, including fire safety building features
- Your process for maintaining and testing any fire safety equipment, emergency power systems, and medical gas and vacuum systems
- Your compliance with *Life Safety Code* requirements
- Actions necessary for you to address any identified compliance deficiencies

Life Safety Code surveyor: In hospitals and critical access hospitals, as well as ambulatory health care settings, a *Life Safety Code* surveyor participates in the LS Session part of the survey—for one or several days, depending on the size of the organization. This person knows the LS requirements inside and out, leads the document review, and conducts the Facility Orientation and the *Life Safety Code* Building Assessment.

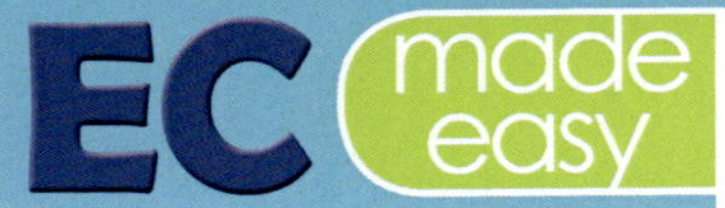

Although the building assessment is mainly about compliance and observation (*see* below), the surveyor routinely reviews life safety–related documents before starting the assessment.

Life Safety Code *Building Assessment:* The *Life Safety Code* Building Assessment is a central part of the survey. In hospitals, critical access hospitals, and ambulatory health care settings, the *Life Safety Code* surveyor leads this assessment; in other settings, it's led by a member of the survey team. The assessment looks at the following:

- Critical pressure relationship areas
- Hazardous areas (soiled linen rooms, trash collection rooms, kitchen)
- Required fire separations and/or smoke barriers
- Exits (number and locations) and corridor clutter
- Equipment and systems (fire alarm, emergency power systems, medical gas and vacuum components)
- Trash and linen chutes
- Fire pump and generators
- Exits and illumination
- Lab roof exhausts
- Fire and smoke doors

Above-the-ceiling inspections: In all settings, the surveyor systematically conducts "above the ceiling" inspections to identify any structure deficiencies related to fire and smoke walls, walls around fire-rated enclosures, corridor walls, ceilings, and fireproofing on structural components like columns or beams and around metal ductwork (based on manufacturers' recommendations). Be ready to explain what types of fire-stopping materials are being used and what training has occurred for the facility staff and contractors. You might also be asked to identify any infection control issues with removing ceiling tiles to determine where this is appropriate and identify where immunocompromised patients may be located (*see* Chapter 9). This will be done prior to the start of the building assessment.

KEY CONCEPT

The Survey Analysis for Evaluating Risk™ (SAFER™) Matrix

Implicit in the survey process is the goal of minimizing or eliminating risk. However, the immediacy of the risk posed by noncompliance varies among standards and EPs and within the context of the organization's compliance. A nonfunctioning sprinkler system, for example, presents a more immediately dangerous situation than a leadership vacancy. Because of this, The Joint Commission created the SAFER matrix to more appropriately classify different risk levels posed by noncompliance with standards.

SAFER matrix: Each observation recorded by a surveyor will be plotted on the Survey Analysis for Evaluating Risk™ (SAFER™) matrix according to the likelihood to cause harm (low, moderate, high) to patients, staff, and/or visitors, as well as the scope (limited, pattern, widespread) at which the Requirement for Improvement (RFI) was observed. This can help your organization focus its improvement efforts. Any RFIs placed in the upper right regions (dark orange or red boxes) of the matrix pose a greater risk in terms of the number of persons potentially affected or the severity of that risk. They require extra documentation in the Evidence of Standards Compliance (ESC), as described in the following section. *See* the "Survey Analysis for Evaluating Risk™ (SAFER™) Matrix Resources" sidebar on page 193 for information to help your organization better understand the SAFER matrix process.

Immediate Threat to Health or Safety

Situations considered an "Immediate Threat to Health or Safety" cause immediate risk and must be addressed promptly. They're also referred to as an "Immediate Threat to Life" (ITL), and are plotted on the SAFER matrix in the top row.

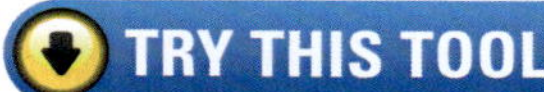

The SAFER™ Matrix
Use this tool to plot out any self-identified compliance issues to help focus attention on areas in most need for improvement. EC, EM, and LS examples are included on the second page in this tool.

in other words

Immediate Threat to Health or Safety
A situation that poses an immediate risk of serious adverse effects on the health or safety of a patient. This is identified on site by a surveyor during survey. Also known as *Immediate Threat to Life (ITL)*.

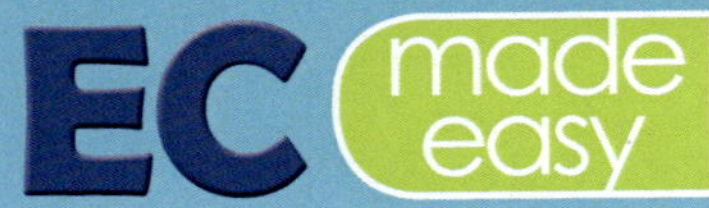

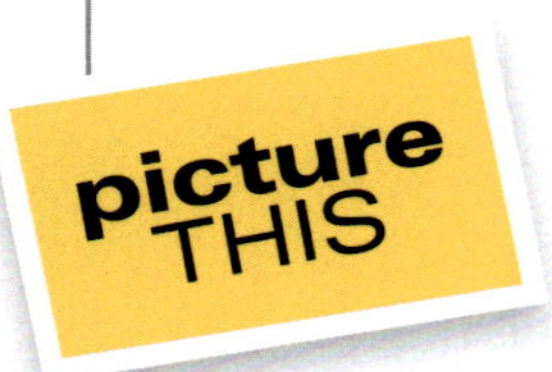

The SAFER Matrix

Each observation reported by a surveyor will be plotted on the SAFER matrix according to the risk level of the finding—that is, the *likelihood of the finding to cause harm* to patients, staff, and/or visitors and the *scope* at which the RFI was observed. As the risk level of a finding or an observation increases, the placement of the standard and EP moves from the bottom left corner (lowest risk level) to the upper right corner (highest risk level).

Situations leading to an ITL finding: In the environment of care, difficulties within the following important systems and situations can lead to an ITL finding:

- Emergency generator (failure, lack of, poor placement)
- Sprinkler system (failure, inadequate testing and maintenance)
- Fire alarm system (failure, inadequate testing and maintenance)
- Main medical gas panel (failure, not monitored)
- Exits (compromised, lack of, doors not operable)

Survey Analysis for Evaluating Risk™ (SAFER™) Matrix Resources

The Survey Analysis for Evaluating Risk (SAFER) is a transformative approach for identifying and communicating risk levels associated with deficiencies cited during surveys. The additional information related to risk provided by the SAFER matrix helps organizations prioritize and focus corrective actions. The Joint Commission has developed a portal to highlight the many SAFER resources available. Visit the portal at www.jointcommission.org/safer to:

- Help your organization understand the overall SAFER concept
- Identify key elements of the SAFER matrix process
- Learn how the SAFER matrix is scored in the field
- Understand ESC requirements and sustaining corrective actions
- Utilize ongoing educational opportunities

The portal has the following helpful resources to choose from:

- Resources (topic library items, PowerPoints, infographics, templates, etc.)
- Videos (SAFER matrix demos and frequently asked questions)
- SAFER webinar replays
- Blogs
- Podcasts
- Joint Commission online articles
- Joint Commission requirements from *Perspectives*

Responses to an ITL finding: If certain problems with these systems are discovered during survey, your organization may advance to an ITL recommendation. The surveyor will notify your CEO and Joint Commission headquarters of the ITL finding and, if your organization uses deemed status, The Joint Commission will notify CMS after confirming the threat. Your organization will then have up to 72 hours to eliminate the risk completely, or implement interim life safety measures (ILSMs) to abate life safety risks (*see* Chapter 7 and Chapter 9) and/or other measures to abate other risks until they can be completely eliminated.

smart questions:

Has your organization ever had an ITL finding? What are the details?

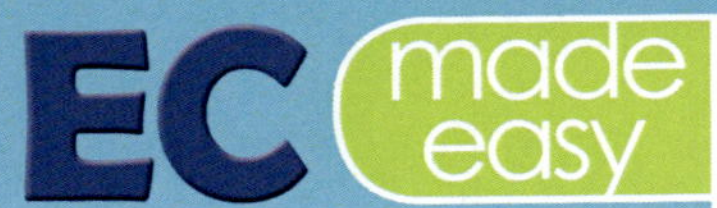

in other words

Requirement for Improvement (RFI)

A recommendation that an organization must address in its Evidence of Standards Compliance (ESC) in order to retain accreditation.

Survey-Related Plan for Improvement (SPFI)

A structural environment of care or life safety deficiency that resulted in a Requirement for Improvement (RFI), but cannot be resolved within the 60 days evidence of standards compliance. The SPFI documents the deficiency and manages the resolution within the Statement of Conditions™.

smart questions:

What environment of care, emergency management, or life safety RFIs did your organization get in the last survey?

Decision Rules

Specific problematic situations may warrant a recommendation for Preliminary Denial of Accreditation, or The Joint Commission may make a decision known as Accreditation with Follow-up Survey.

- **What kind of situations?** Some examples of these situations include lack of facility or individual licensure, or failure to respond to identified *Life Safety Code* deficiencies.
- **What if you're noncompliant?** If your organization is noncompliant with these types of situations, you must follow up with an ESC submission (*see* page 195).

The ACC chapter in the *CAMs* and on E-dition describes this process in greater detail.

KEY CONCEPT

After the Survey

Shortly after your survey is completed, an accreditation report will be posted to your organization's *Joint Commission Connect*™ extranet site (*see* the sidebar "*Joint Commission Connect*™" on page 195). The report summarizes survey results in the SAFER matrix, then provides details on individual findings.

Requirements for Improvement (RFIs)

Be prepared: Most organizations receive Requirements for Improvement (RFIs). An RFI means that surveyors found that your organization doesn't comply with a particular standard because noncompliance with one or more EPs was observed. All RFIs must be addressed within 60 days from the last day of survey before an accreditation decision can be made. Any structural environment of care or life safety deficiencies that cannot be corrected within the 60 days must be managed as a Survey-Related Plan for Improvement (SPFI) within the organization's Statement of Conditions™ (SOC). An SPFI must request a time-limited waiver (TLW) for the additional time that the organization will need to resolve the deficiency. The organization must have a Joint Commission–approved TLW at time of submission of their ESC.

Evidence of Standards Compliance (ESC)

For each RFI, your organization must submit an Evidence of Standards Compliance (ESC) report. There are two types of ESCs:

- **Corrective ESC:** This explains what actions your organization took to bring itself into compliance. It must do the following:
  - *Assign accountability.* The ESC must identify *who* is ultimately responsible for the corrective actions. In addition, if the finding falls in the higher levels of the SAFER matrix, you must also document leadership's role in the actions. (These RFIs will also be flagged for review in ensuing surveys.)
  - *Correct the noncompliance.* Describe *what* actions you took and *when* to correct noncompliance. Again, if the finding rates high on the matrix, you must also document any preventive analysis of what went wrong that will help to achieve and maintain compliance.
  - *Ensure sustained compliance.* The ESC has been expanded to focus on sustaining the improvements. Describe what procedures or activities you will use to monitor compliance with the EP, the frequency of the monitoring activities, the data that will be collected from these activities, and how and to whom these data will be reported.

in other words

Evidence of Standards Compliance (ESC)

A report that a surveyed organization must submit within 60 days after a survey in which it receives a Requirement for Improvement (RFI) for an accreditation requirement. The report must detail actions taken to bring the organization into compliance with each requirement, or explain why the organization believes it's in compliance. The report has to address compliance at the element of performance (EP) level.

smart questions:

Who is your Joint Commission account executive?

Joint Commission Connect™

Whether you're applying for Joint Commission accreditation or are already accredited, you need to keep your accreditation information up to date. This is done via your organization's *Joint Commission Connect™* extranet site. *Joint Commission Connect* is a secure extranet website intended only for organizations accredited or certified by The Joint Commission. It contains many useful resources about the survey process and tools for continuous compliance. It's also how you exchange important and confidential information with The Joint Commission. Each organization is responsible for designating who has access to *Joint Commission Connect*. If you're an accredited organization, or an organization seeking Joint Commission accreditation, you can contact your account executive for access assistance.

Account executive: This person serves as the primary contact between your organization and The Joint Commission. Your account executive coordinates survey planning and handles policies, procedures, accreditation issues or services, and inquiries throughout the accreditation cycle. Your account executive is listed on your *Joint Commission Connect* home page.

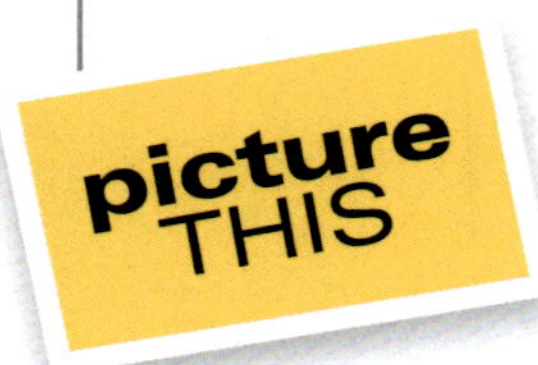

SAFER Matrix Follow-Up

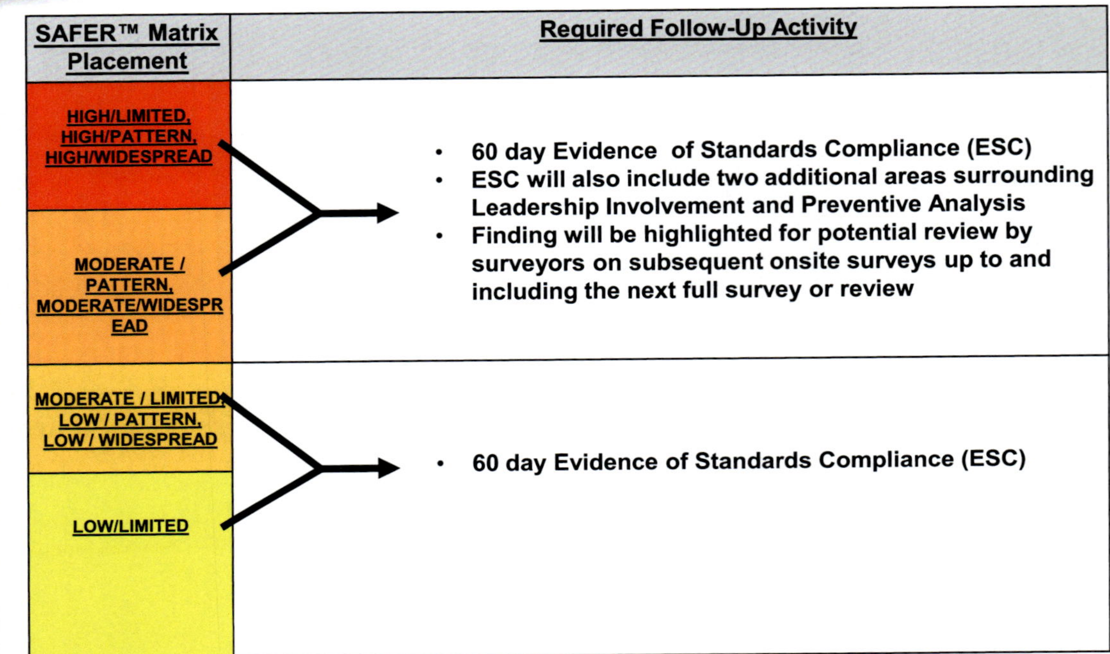

The SAFER™ matrix information provides a representation of possible required ESC follow-up activities for Requirements for Improvement (RFIs) of varying risk levels.

- **Clarifying process:** This is used when your organization believes it was compliant at the time of the survey and must be completed and submitted within 10 days of the receipt of the final survey report. The intent of the clarification is to demonstrate compliance at the time of survey specific to survey observations that organizations feel they were in compliance with. A few things to keep in mind about clarifying ESCs:
- Challenging a surveyor's observation doesn't automatically remove an RFI. Keep working on a corrective ESC until you hear back from The Joint Commission.
- You'll need to show proof supporting your claim that you were compliant and when you were. You must show you met

the standard at the time of survey—not during or immediately after.

- Any required documents that are not available at the time of survey will no longer be eligible for the clarification process. These RFIs will become action items in the post-survey corrective ESC process.
- Clerical errors in the report will no longer be eligible for the clarification process. The Joint Commission will work with the organization to ensure that the report is accurate, and the corrected RFIs will become action items in the post-survey corrective ESC process.

Time-Limited Waivers (TLWs)

The SPFI process includes time-limited waivers (TLWs). A TLW is required if the scheduled completion date for resolving the deficiency will exceed 60 days. A TLW is a formal request from a health care organization for additional time to resolve an environment of care or a life safety deficiency. A TLW must be submitted within 45 days from the end of survey. When an organization requests a TLW, The Joint Commission evaluates the request and, for those organizations that use accreditation for deemed status purposes, forwards it to the appropriate CMS regional office within the required 60-day period. If the TLW is acceptable, The Joint Commission will update the organiza-

in other words

time-limited waiver (TLW)

A formal request for additional time to resolve an environment of care or a life safety deficiency. As part of the application and approval process, the organization will work with The Joint Commission and the appropriate US Centers for Medicare & Medicaid Services regional office to establish a scheduled completion date (SCD) for corrective actions.

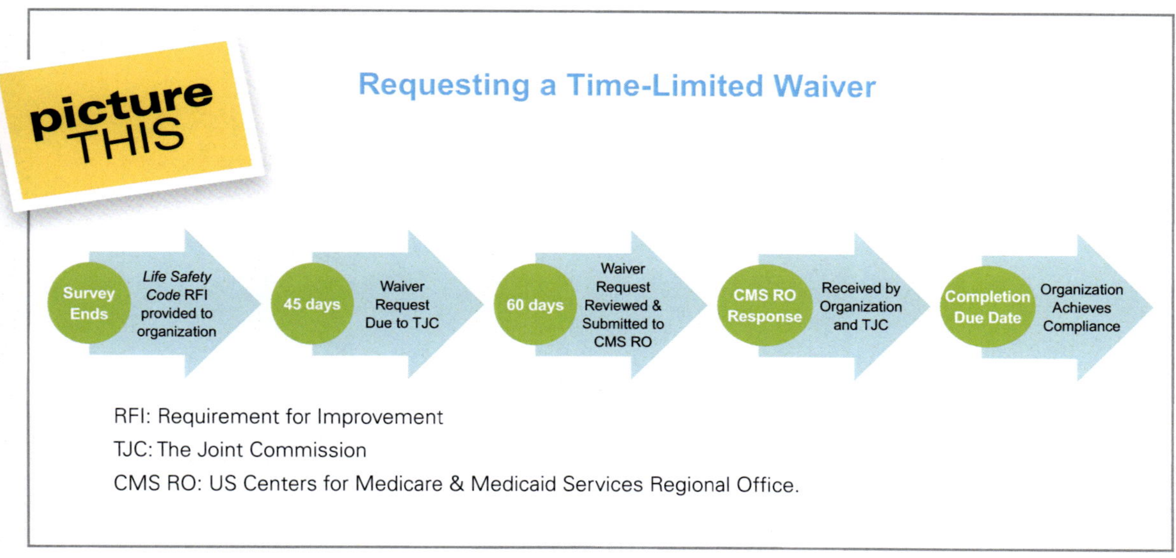

RFI: Requirement for Improvement

TJC: The Joint Commission

CMS RO: US Centers for Medicare & Medicaid Services Regional Office.

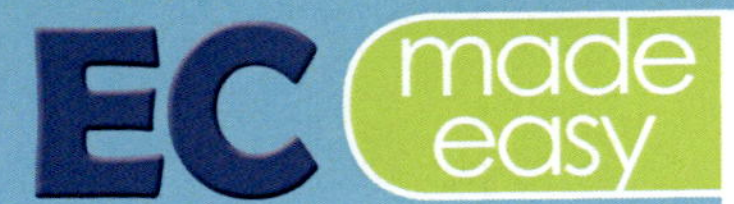

tion's scheduled completion date and approve the TLW request as well as the corresponding SPFI.

Achieving Accreditation

When your organization achieves accreditation, The Joint Commission will send you a certificate. You should receive it two to three weeks after the decision. For details on the use of the certificate, refer to the ACC chapter of the *CAM*s or the publicity kit available on the Joint Commission website.

KEY CONCEPT

Continuous Compliance

Because compliance with Joint Commission standards is a measure of patient safety and quality of care, it should be consistently high and continuously monitored through tracers and performance improvement programs.

Intracycle Monitoring (ICM) Profile

The Joint Commission offers a suite of tools to help you maintain compliance between surveys: the Intracycle Monitoring (ICM) Profile. Through your secure *Joint Commission Connect* extranet site, you can access your organization's ICM Profile. The profile includes your accreditation status information, major risk areas, and resources.

Your risk areas: Your ICM Profile identifies high-risk areas by program and labels them with a special **R** icon. These are evaluated based on the proximity to the patient, the severity of potential harm, and the number of patients exposed to the risk. They're categorized according to The Joint Commission's National Patient Safety Goals, program-specific risk areas, and RFIs from your most recent survey.

On-site ICM: You may also request an on-site ICM survey and ask for surveyors to address specific current needs, such as medical staff or environment of care or *Life Safety Code* issues, so the composition of the surveyor team will match your needs.

in other words

Intracycle Monitoring (ICM)

A process that helps accredited organizations maintain continuous compliance through a self-assessment of high-risk areas and related standards. It involves use of the organization's ICM Profile available on the organization's *Joint Commission Connect*™ extranet site.

Focused Standards Assessment (FSA)

One major component of the ICM Profile is the Focused Standards Assessment (FSA). Your accredited organization must complete this self-assessment activity every year between Joint Commission surveys (unless you're an office-based surgery program). You can choose to do it yourself or ask for help. It scores the same way surveyors do during an on-site survey, identifies areas of noncompliance, and requires a Plan of Action (POA) for any RFI. Additionally, when completing the FSA, organizations have the option of making SAFER scope and likelihood to harm designations, resulting in a SAFER matrix upon completion of the FSA.

Structural environment of care and life safety deficiencies that cannot be completed within the 60 days POA are required to manage those deficiencies as a Plan for Improvement (PFI) in their Statement of Conditions (SOC). The PFI unique identification number should be referenced within your ICM submission. The FSA is intended to help organizations work the standards into everyday operations. You're required to complete an FSA assessment for all high-risk standards, as labeled with the icon, although you can complete an assessment of *all* EPs with the online tool. The FSA tool is accessible throughout the accreditation cycle in the ICM Profile.

Tie to the Statement of Conditions: POA is required for any structural EC and LS deficiencies that cannot be completed within 60 days. You are required to manage those deficiencies as a PFI in your SOC. Reference the PFI unique identification number within your ICM submission.

Impact of the FSA on accreditation: The FSA doesn't affect your organization's accreditation status unless (1) you don't participate in the FSA, or (2) the FSA identifies an ITL and a special survey is conducted.

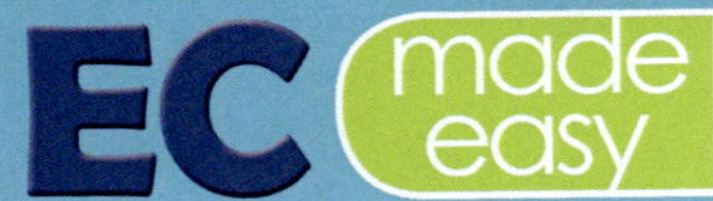

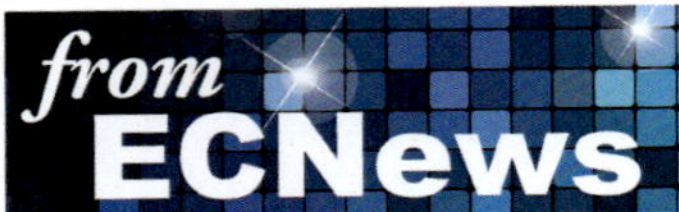

Tracing the Environment of Care

Your organization can capitalize on the benefits of tracer methodology by conducting "mock tracers"—practice tracers meant to simulate an actual tracer. . . . Performing environment of care (EC) mock tracers is not difficult, although the process is slightly different than the process for performing tracers that assess clinical issues. During EC mock tracers, the individual conducting the tracer—the "mock surveyor"—must focus on organizational systems and processes specifically related to the physical environment rather than examine the care, treatment, and services patients receive.

Subjects for an EC mock tracer include systems and processes that relate to safety, security, hazardous materials and waste, fire safety, utilities, and medical equipment as well as emergency management and life safety. For example, an EC mock tracer might examine the security of pharmaceuticals throughout an organization, the installation and maintenance of a heating, ventilating, and air-conditioning (HVAC) system, or an organization's emergency preparedness and emergency exercise efforts.

—excerpted from "Tracing the Environment of Care: An Essential Approach to Identifying Safety Risks and Compliance Issues," *Environment of Care® News*, March 2011

COLLABORATION: Accreditation professionals, consider implementing a mock tracer program if you don't already have one. Mock tracers simulate tracers like those surveyors use. They can help you assess compliance issues on an ongoing basis and come up with plans to address them. Plus, tracers get staff used to the on-site survey process and what interaction with a surveyor will be like. Most importantly, tracers support continuous compliance. Facilities directors, you can work with the tracer team on tracers focused on the physical environment.

TOOLS OF THE TRADE

- Required EC Documentation Checklist
- Tracer Questions and the Mock Tracer Form
- On-Site Survey Readiness Checklist
- The SAFER™ Matrix

Resources

The published and online resources below are provided to help you find more information from The Joint Commission and Joint Commission Resources (JCR) on the topics covered in this book.*

Accreditation Manuals

The Joint Commission. *2017 Comprehensive Accreditation Manuals*. Oak Brook, IL: Joint Commission Resources, 2017. http://www.jcrinc.com/2017-comprehensive-accreditation-manuals/ [Published annually. Updated semi-annually.]

- *Comprehensive Accreditation Manual for Ambulatory Care*
- *Comprehensive Accreditation Manual for Behavioral Health Care*
- *Comprehensive Accreditation Manual for Critical Access Hospitals*
- *Comprehensive Accreditation Manual for Home Care*
- *Comprehensive Accreditation Manual for Hospitals*
- *Comprehensive Accreditation Manual for Laboratory and Point-of-Care Testing*
- *Comprehensive Accreditation Manual for Nursing Care Centers*

Standards are also available via E-dition®.

JCR Periodicals

The Joint Commission. *Environment of Care® News*. http://www.jcrinc.com/environment-of-care-news/ [Published monthly.]

The Joint Commission. *The Joint Commission Journal on Quality and Patient Safety®*. http://www.jointcommissionjournal.com [Published monthly.]

* All online resources were active at the time of publication of this book.

The Joint Commission. *The Joint Commission Perspectives®*. http://www.jcrinc.com/the-joint-commission-perspectives/ [Published monthly; e-version free to accredited organizations.]

The Joint Commission. *The Joint Commission: The Source™*. http://www.jcrinc.com/the-source/ [Published monthly.]

JCR Books

Books listed below are available as hard copy or eBook versions unless otherwise noted.

The Joint Commission. *Environment of Care®: Essentials for Health Care*. Oak Brook, IL: Joint Commission Resources, published annually. http://www.jcrinc.com/2017-environment-of -care-essentials-for-health-care/

The Joint Commission. *Environment of Care® Crosswalk*. Oak Brook, IL: Joint Commission Resources, published annually. http://www.jcrinc.com/environment-of-care-2017-crosswalk/

The Joint Commission. *Environment of Care® Risk Assessment*, 3rd Edition. Oak Brook, IL: Joint Commission Resources, 2017. http://www.jcrinc.com/environment-of-care -risk-assessment-3rd-edition/

The Joint Commission. *Emergency Management in Health Care: An All-Hazards Approach*, Third Edition. Oak Brook, IL: Joint Commission Resources, 2016. http://www.jcrinc.com /emergency-management-in-health-care-third-edition/

The Joint Commission. *The Joint Commission Big Book of Checklists*. Oak Brook, IL: Joint Commission Resources, 2016. http://www.jcrinc.com/the-joint-commission-big-book-of -checklists/ [Published July 2016.]

The Joint Commission. *Toolkit for New Accreditation Professionals*, 2nd Edition. Oak Brook, IL: Joint Commission Resources, 2017. http://www.jcrinc.com/toolkit-for-new -accreditation-professionals-2nd-edition/

The Joint Commission. *Infection Prevention and Control Issues in the Environment of Care*, Third Edition. Oak Brook, IL: Joint Commission Resources, 2017. http://www.jcrinc.com/infection-prevention-and-control-issues-in-the-environment-of-care-3rd-edition/

The Joint Commission. *Planning, Design, and Construction of Health Care Facilities*, Revised Third Edition. Oak Brook, IL: Joint Commission Resources, 2017. http://www.jcrinc.com/planning-design-and-construction-of-health-care-facilities-third-edition/

Online Portals

The Joint Commission. *Emergency Management Resources*. Oak Brook, IL: Joint Commission Resources, 2017. https://www.jointcommission.org/emergency_management.aspx

The Joint Commission. *The Infection Prevention and HAI Portal*. Oak Brook, IL: Joint Commission Resources, 2017. https://www.jointcommission.org/hai.aspx

The Joint Commission. *Patient Safety*. Oak Brook, IL: Joint Commission Resources, 2017. https://www.jointcommission.org/topics/patient_safety.aspx

The Joint Commission. *Life Safety Code Information & Resources*. Oak Brook, IL. Joint Commission Resources, 2017. https://www.jointcommission.org/life_safety_code_information_resources/

The Joint Commission. *The Physical Environment Portal*. Oak Brook, IL: Joint Commission Resources, 2017. https://www.jointcommission.org/topics/the_physical_environment.aspx

The Joint Commission. *Survey Analysis for Evaluating Risk™ (SAFER™) Matrix Resources*. Oak Brook, IL: Joint Commission Resources, 2017. https://www.jointcommission.org/topics/safer_matrix_resources.aspx

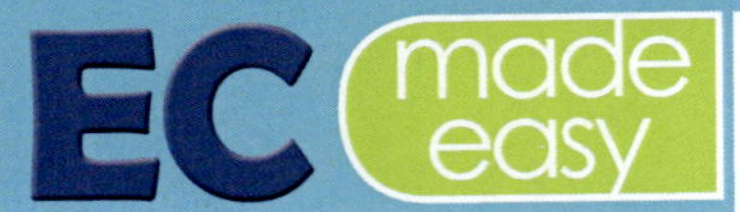

The Joint Commission. *Workplace Violence Prevention Resources*. Oak Brook, IL: Joint Commission Resources, 2017. https://www.jointcommission.org/workplace_violence.aspx

The Joint Commission Enterprise Content Library
The Joint Commission. *The Joint Commission Enterprise Content Library*. Oakbrook Terrace, IL: The Joint Commission, 2017. https://www.jointcommission.org/enterprise_content_library_index/ [updated quarterly]